T0234527

Promoting Healthy and Active Aging

This book demonstrates the efficacy of a multidisciplinary intervention strategy for promoting active and healthy aging, with the assistance of dedicated technological resources.

Taking an applied approach, this book promotes active and healthy aging through the implementation of an intervention model based on the comprehensive geriatric approach (AGA). The proposed AGA model, entitled AGA@4life, is based on a holistic and multidisciplinary individual assessment protocol, with the consequent design and implementation of intervention strategies tailored to each individual, aimed at preventing frailty and functional, cognitive, and social decline of the elderly. Intervention actions focus on personalized exercise programs, nutrition education, cognitive stimulation, co-morbidity monitoring, therapeutic counseling, and overall promotion of well-being.

This book will be of interest to researchers, professionals, and students working in aging and health, gerontology, and preventative and holistic approaches to well-being.

Telmo Pereira is Professor and Head of the Physiology Department and Coordinator of the Labinsaúde Research Center, Polytechnic Institute of Coimbra, Coimbra Health School, Coimbra, Portugal.

Promoting Healthy and Active Aging

A Multidisciplinary Approach

Edited by
Telmo Pereira

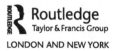
Routledge
Taylor & Francis Group

LONDON AND NEW YORK

First published 2022
by Routledge
2 Park Square, Milton Park, Abingdon, Oxon OX14 4RN

and by Routledge
52 Vanderbilt Avenue, New York, NY 10017

Routledge is an imprint of the Taylor & Francis Group, an informa business

© 2022 selection and editorial matter, **Telmo Pereira**; individual chapters, the contributors

The right of **Telmo Pereira** to be identified as the author of the editorial material, and of the authors for their individual chapters, has been asserted in accordance with sections 77 and 78 of the Copyright, Designs and Patents Act 1988.

All rights reserved. No part of this book may be reprinted or reproduced or utilised in any form or by any electronic, mechanical, or other means, now known or hereafter invented, including photocopying and recording, or in any information storage or retrieval system, without permission in writing from the publishers.

Trademark notice: Product or corporate names may be trademarks or registered trademarks, and are used only for identification and explanation without intent to infringe.

British Library Cataloguing-in-Publication Data
A catalogue record for this book is available from the British Library

Library of Congress Cataloging-in-Publication Data
A catalog record has been requested for this book

ISBN: 978-1-032-05727-9 (hbk)
ISBN: 978-1-032-10424-9 (pbk)
ISBN: 978-1-003-21527-1 (ebk)

DOI: 10.4324/9781003215271

Typeset in Baskerville
by KnowledgeWorks Global Ltd.

Contents

List of figures   vii
List of tables   ix
List of contributors   x

1 **A multidisciplinary approach to promote an active
   and healthy aging: The AGA@4life model**   1
   TELMO PEREIRA

2 **Promoting functional ability and falls prevention:
   Strategies for healthy aging**   9
   ANABELA CORREIA MARTINS, DANIELA GUIA, AND MARINA SARAIVA

3 **Physical exercise applied to older people**   24
   INÊS CIPRIANO AND TELMO PEREIRA

4 **BrainAnswer platform: Biosignals acquisition for
   monitoring of physical and cardiac conditions of
   older people**   36
   JOÃO VALENTE, VERONIKA KOZLOVA, AND TELMO PEREIRA

5 **Nutrition in aging**   56
   MARIA HELENA LOUREIRO

6 **Evaluation of indoor air quality and its importance
   for health and wellness promotion in the older adult**   65
   ANA FERREIRA, ANTÓNIO LOUREIRO, AND SILVIA SECO

 7 **Pharmacological treatment and the polymedicated
    older adult**   83
    ANA PAULA FONSECA AND VERA GALINHA

 8 **The effect of auditory training in the older adult's lives**   90
    CARLA MATOS SILVA, CAROLINA FERNANDES, AND CLARA ROCHA

 9 **Age-associated changes in cholesterol metabolism
    cardiovascular risk and exercise effect on lipid profile**   99
    ISABEL SILVA, MARIANA CLEMENTE, CARLA FERREIRA,
    ANA MARGARIDA SILVA, ANTÓNIO GABRIEL, TELMO PEREIRA,
    AND ARMANDO CASEIRO

10 **Impact of a multidisciplinary intervention program
    on skeletal muscle in the older adult**   114
    RUTE SANTOS

11 **Structural and functional changes of the aging heart**   124
    JOAQUIM CASTANHEIRA AND TELMO PEREIRA

12 **Modulators and determinants of arterial aging
    in the older adult**   130
    TATIANA COSTA AND TELMO PEREIRA

13 **Hepatic characterization of the senior population
    and its relationship with polymedication**   141
    RUTE SANTOS

14 **Cognitive function and aging**   149
    TELMO PEREIRA

    Index   161

Figures

1.1 Dimensions and subdimensions of the comprehensive
    geriatric approach   3
4.1 Demographics data platform implementation interface.
    Information to the participant about the demographic
    questionnaire and clinical situation of some parameters.
    The participant may continue or give up and the
    response time is not limited. Questionnaire response
    with no limited response time. The screen is fullscreen   40
4.2 Platform interface for IPAQ placement. Information
    to the participant about physical activity questionnaire.
    Response time is not limited. The screen is fullscreen   41
4.3 Platform interface for 300 seconds ECG acquisition time.
    Performing ECG Signal Collection: Information on the
    procedures to be taken into account during ECG
    registration and the conditions that must be observed
    during collection. The participant may continue or
    give up and the response time is not limited. ECG
    registration with fixed duration of 300 seconds.
    Registration ends with a thank you. The system
    returns a message if the data was submitted correctly   41
4.4 Interface for selection and configuration of equipment
    to be used   42
4.5 BrainAnswer Client   42
4.6 Raw data Treatment: (a) Acquired ECG signal, top graph.
    (b) Filtered signal and location/marking with R wave
    points, middle graph. (c) Heart rate estimation,
    graph below   44

4.7 Display of participant (34) left side and participant (3) right side signals. The graphs above correspond to the raw signal, the middle signals correspond to the filtered ECG signal and the R wave markers (yellow dots) are calculated by the algorithm. The graph below corresponds to the variation of each participant's heartbeat   45

4.8 HRV time parameters and histogram nni (a) participant (34), older adult, left side and (b) participant (3) young, right side   47

4.9 Spectral result of HRV parameters (a) of the older participant and (b) of the younger participant   49

4.10 Parameters obtained from nonlinear analysis. SD1, SD2, and SD1/SD2 ratios obtained from Poincaré plot   51

Tables

3.1 Schema for the prescription of exercise in the older
  adult with chronic diseases   31
4.1 Comparison of HRV time parameters for older adult
  and young participant   48
4.2 Comparison of HRV frequency parameters for older
  adult and young participant   50
4.3 Summary display of the IPAQ classification for
  physical activity. Left table represents the absolute and
  relative frequencies according to group (old versus young)
  and level of physical activity (high, moderate, and low).
  Right table depicts the weekly averages for hours of
  exercise (Avg HE), number of days of exercise (Avg DE)
  and sitting hours (Avg HS)   52
6.1 Effects of environmental pollutants on health   67
6.2 Average concentration of environmental parameters   71
6.3 Average concentration of environmental parameters
  by interior space evaluated   72
6.4 Average pollutant concentration, temperature, and
  relative humidity, depending on the time of measurement
  for indoor and outdoor   73
6.5 Relationship between pollutants and temperature and
  relative humidity   74
6.6 Presence of symptoms/pathologies in the older
  adult day center   75
10.1 Aging process: biological, psychological, and
  social dimensions   115
10.2 Structural changes resulting from aging and clinical
  manifestations   116
12.1 Determinants of the early vascular aging (EVA)   133
14.1 Additional changes in the aging brain   151

Contributors

Armando Caseiro is a professor of the Laboratory Biomedical Sciences Department of the Coimbra Health School, Polytechnic Institute of Coimbra

Joaquim Castanheira is a professor of the Clinical Physiology Department of the Coimbra Health School, Polytechnic Institute of Coimbra

Inês Cipriano holds a Bachelor's degree in Clinical Physiology, Master in Sports Sciences, Polytechnic Institute of Coimbra

Mariana Clemente holds a Bachelor's degree in Laboratory Biomedical Sciences from the Polytechnic Institute of Coimbra

Anabela Correia Martins is a professor of the Physiotherapy Department of the Coimbra Health School, Polytechnic Institute of Coimbra

Tatiana Costa holds a Bachelor's degree in Clinical Physiology, Polytechnic Institute of Coimbra

Carolina Fernandes holds a Bachelor's degree in Audiology from the Polytechnic Institute of Coimbra

Ana Ferreira is a professor in the Environmental Health Department of the Coimbra Health School, Vice-President of the Polytechnic Institute of Coimbra

Carla Ferreira holds a Bachelor's degree in Laboratory Biomedical Sciences from the Polytechnic Institute of Coimbra

Ana Paula Fonseca is a professor of the Pharmacy Department of the Coimbra Health School, Polytechnic Institute of Coimbra

António Gabriel is a professor of the Laboratory Biomedical Sciences Department of the Coimbra Health School, Polytechnic Institute of Coimbra

Vera Galinha holds a Masters in Pharmacy, Polytechnic Institute of Coimbra

Daniela Guia holds a Bachelor's degree in Physiotherapy, Polytechnic Institute of Coimbra

Veronika Kozlova is a professor of the Exact Sciences Department of the Polytechnic Institute of Castelo-Branco

António Loureiro holds a Bachelor's degree in Environmental Health, Polytechnic Institute of Coimbra

Rute Santos is a professor of the Medical Imaging and Radiotherapy Department of the Coimbra Health School, Polytechnic Institute of Coimbra

Marina Saraiva holds a Masters in Physiotherapy, Polytechnic Institute of Coimbra

Sílvia Seco holds a Bachelor's degree in Environmental Health, Polytechnic Institute of Coimbra

Ana Margarida Silva holds a Bachelor's degree in Laboratory Biomedical Sciences, Polytechnic Institute of Coimbra

Carla Matos Silva is a professor of the Audiology Department of the Coimbra Health School, Polytechnic Institute of Coimbra

Clara Rocha is a professor of the Exact Sciences Department of the Coimbra Health School, Polytechnic Institute of Coimbra

Isabel Silva holds a Bachelor's degree in Laboratory Biomedical Sciences, Polytechnic Institute of Coimbra

João Valente is a professor of the Exact Sciences Department of the Polytechnic Institute of Castelo-Branco. CEO at the BrainAnswer, Lda., Castelo-Branco, Portugal

Maria Helena Vieira Soares Loureiro is a professor of the Dietetics and Nutrition Department of the Coimbra Health School, Polytechnic Institute of Coimbra

1 A multidisciplinary approach to promote an active and healthy aging
The AGA@4life model

Telmo Pereira

Introduction

Population aging is today a major social and economic problem, with growth in the European Union at a rate of over 2 million people over 60 years per year[1]. Increasing average life expectancy and declining birth rates are drivers of a demographic transformation process that creates a set of new challenges regarding the insertion of the older adult in the society, the quality and life expectancy of the older adult, the sustainability of health systems, health and social security, and the labor market[2]. On the other hand, demographic pressure on specialized care institutions for these populations will also pose operational problems, which could compromise the quality of the services provided and the adequacy of supply to all those in need of such support[3]. Recognizing these challenges is crucial to the development and implementation of policies and strategic actions that value the role of the older adult, promote their health and well-being, and contribute to their involvement and participation in the community[4].

The challenge

Demographic aging presents different challenges to modern societies, namely: (1) at the public administration level, concerning the insertion of the older adult in society, the quality and life expectancy, and the sustainability of health systems; (2) at the level of caregivers, in view of the operational problems that may arise from excessive demographic pressure, with a foreseeable impact on the quality of services and the adequacy of supply; (3) on academia, particularly in the area of Health Sciences, by the need to adapt curricula to the clinical complexity of these populations, in the areas that mediate health promotion and disease prevention, diagnosis, treatment, and

DOI: 10.4324/9781003215271-1

rehabilitation; and (4) at the societal level, for the humanistic purpose of guaranteeing individual dignity. On the other hand, the biological, psychological, and social context of the older adult is admittedly very particular. First, the intrinsic physiological processes of aging are a fundamental determinant of the effectiveness of initiatives aimed at promoting active and healthy aging[3,4]. In fact, this population is at higher risk for deficiencies acquired at various levels, cognitive decline, hospitalization, or other forms of institutionalization as a consequence of illness or the inherent therapeutic process[5-7]. On the other hand, the clinical context of the older adult is marked by enormous complexity, with the coexistence of several chronic diseases, often clinically occult (Iceberg phenomenon), and with the consequent polypharmacy representing an added challenge[5], and furthermore with insidious loss of functionality, frailty, risk of falls[8], and increased risk of mortality[9]. In particular, the risk of falls has motivated the development of screening and prevention technology resources, such as the innovative FallSensing system[10].

The answer

The answer to this first-line problem will necessarily have to be an individualized, multidimensional, and interdisciplinary approach, which forms the root of the comprehensive geriatric approach (AGA). Marjory Warren proposed this model in the late thirties of the last century, assuming it to be an answer to the complexity and multiplicity of problems presented by the older adult[11], so this approach is one of the cornerstones in geriatric care. This model is a multidisciplinary process, based on the diagnostic-intervention continuum, by identifying the physical, mental, and social limitations and disabilities of the older adult, and implementing a coordinated and individualized intervention plan, aiming at maximizing health during aging[12,13]. Thus, care is directed beyond traditional clinical management, incorporating physical, cognitive, affective, social, environmental, and even financial and spiritual components, which are crucial for a holistic welfare perspective[14] (see Figure 1.1). AGA has traditionally been based on the premise that a systematic assessment of the older adult by a multidisciplinary team enables the optimization of aging management strategies, leading to better health outcomes, health and well-being promotion, and valuing the participation of the older adult in the community[15,16].

In terms of formal structure, AGA is very heterogeneous and flexible. Its components may differ depending on the team applying it

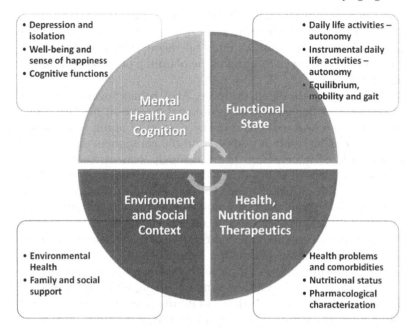

- Depression and isolation
- Well-being and sense of happiness
- Cognitive functions

Mental Health and Cognition

- Daily life activities – autonomy
- Instrumental daily life activities – autonomy
- Equilibrium, mobility and gait

Functional State

Environment and Social Context

Health, Nutrition and Therapeutics

- Environmental Health
- Family and social support

- Health problems and comorbidities
- Nutritional status
- Pharmacological characterization

Figure 1.1 Dimensions and subdimensions of the comprehensive geriatric approach
Source: (AGA).

and where it is performed. However, despite this apparent diversity, AGA has its own and constant characteristics, such as the fact that it is always multidimensional and uses appropriate instruments to quantify functional capacity and to evaluate psychological and social parameters. Incorporating methods from various disciplines into a single assessment provides a practical and objective means of viewing the older adult as a whole[17].

The effectiveness of this approach has been documented in several clinical studies, particularly in settings where selection of the older adult is appropriate, where diagnostic assessment is translated into an individualized intervention plan implemented by an interdisciplinary team, and where systematic monitoring of results is carried out, with dynamic readjustment of intervention programs in the face of changing individual needs[18–22]. The advantages recognized in this model are: (1) at the individual level, better accuracy of clinical examination, establishment of degree and extent of disability, and identification of older adult at risk of functional decline and (2) at the societal level, the identification of populations at risk, and the potential for use in clinical studies for the assessment of functional capacity and quality of life, and in the planning of public policies for aging[23,24].

Given the accumulated evidence, AGA brings together a set of characteristics that make it instrumental for use in health promotion strategies and well-being in the context of aging. The evaluation of the older adult as a whole, and the consequent definition of a personalized intervention plan, in which elements such as intellectual stimulation, physical activity, multidimensional counseling, and promotion of inclusion are key factors, adjust this approach to uniquely address one of today's most complex and important societal challenges[25-27]. Moreover, the most recent evidence in neuroscientific research has documented the contribution of these elements to brain plasticity and cognitive function optimization[28,29]. On the other hand, the positive effect of a physically active, well-fed, and intellectually stimulated body in promoting well-being is also recognized[30]. These aspects, by themselves, illustrate the need for an action plan based on interdisciplinary teams, whose axis of action comprises the physical, psychological/cognitive, social, and cultural interventions, as well as the systematic monitoring of health, for which the use of digital remote monitoring platforms for physiological and environmental biosignals will play a decisive role[31].

The AGA@4life model

The AGA@4life intervention model was designed to meet the societal challenge of demographic aging. In this sense, an intervention program based on AGA was developed, with the fundamental objective of promoting active and healthy aging. The strategic action of this model focuses on valuing the older adult, promoting health and well-being, independence and autonomy, mobility and the opportunity to contribute to the community.

The intervention plan follows the model foreseen in the AGA conceptual design, thus comprising (1) the constitution of an intervention team and the design of the overall action strategy, and (2) the practical implementation of AGA's fundamental steps[12-14,32]. The Intervention Team has a multidisciplinary composition and is responsible for the design and adaptation of the evaluation/intervention model to be implemented, and for all field tasks necessary to achieve the objectives of the intervention plan. As for the implementation of the AGA model, it comprises six fundamental steps: (1) clinical characterization and diagnostic evaluation of the target population; (2) analysis and discussion of the evaluated cases, within the multidisciplinary team; (3) definition of an individualized and multidisciplinary intervention plan; (4) implementation of the intervention plan, in articulation with the older adult, family, and local agents; (5) monitoring the response to the intervention plan; and (6) discussion of the results by the intervention team, and revision of the intervention plan whenever necessary. Compliance with all these steps is critical to achieving the expected result – maximum health and functionality benefit. The key components to be collected in the evaluation of the older adult are: functional capacity, risk of falls, comorbidity (e.g., cardiovascular, respiratory, metabolic, osteo-articular diseases), cognition (e.g., memory, communication), quality of life and mood, polypharmacy, nutrition, hearing and vision, everyday environmental context, dentition, urinary and fecal continence, sexual function, spirituality, social support, financial concerns, and personal expectations for care. To this end, assessment tools are used that include specifically validated questionnaires for use in the context of AGA and technological resources for objective assessments of the cardiovascular, respiratory, digestive and urinary system, overall health status (blood samples), and the evaluation of the muscular and osteoarticular status. The central nervous system is also studied, with an emphasis on the study of cognitive functions by appropriate methods. The physical and environmental characteristics of the places where the daily life of each older person takes place are also evaluated, with emphasis on the study of air quality and physical barriers to mobility. Intervention plans are tailored to the needs identified in each older individual, focusing on the different dimensions that enhance health benefits. One of the central aspects of intervention plans should be, whenever possible, the application of endogenous resources that additionally contribute to valuing the inclusion of the older adult in the ecosystem in which they live.

An additional aspect in the AGA@4life model is the training of health professionals to work in the geriatric context, with particular emphasis on the dimensions of promoting healthy and active aging. In this sense, an interaction with academia in the health sciences is also recommended in order to advise the readjustment of curricula in graduate and post-graduate programs to include problem-based learning and problem-based research applied to the concrete issues of aging.

Conclusions

The challenges inherent to the demographic changes in the contemporary world call for the development of appropriate and effective responses, which should be based on the recognition of aging as an individual multidimensional and heterogeneous process. The AGA@4life intervention model was developed based on this essential premise, combining a holistic approach to the older adult and the consequent definition of a personalized intervention plan to promote healthy and active aging. This intervention plan is tailored to the individual's concrete needs, implemented by a multidisciplinary and technically qualified team, bringing together diverse elements such as cognitive stimulation, adapted physical activity, multidimensional counseling, and the promotion of inclusion.

These aspects illustrate the need for an action plan based on multidisciplinary teams, articulated with Primary Health Care, and with axes of action including neuropsychological, social and cultural interventions, physical activity and functionality, nutritional optimization, and systematic monitoring of global health, in which the use of digital platforms for remote monitoring of physiological signals can play a decisive role. The creation of friendly and inclusive environments valuing the role of the older adult could be an added feature to promote health and well-being, and contribute to the inclusion and social participation of the older adult.

Key points

- Population aging is a major societal challenge.
- Aging is a multidimensional and heterogeneous process.
- Responses to promoting active and healthy aging should be based on a personalized and multidisciplinary approach.
- The AGA@4life model is an integrated, multidisciplinary, and personalized intervention approach to promote an active and healthy aging.

References

1 World Health Organization (WHO). World report on ageing and health. Ageing and life-course. World Health Organization, 2015.
2 Angeloni S, Borgonovi E. An ageing world and the challenges for a model of sustainable social change. J Manag Dev, 2016; 5(4):464–85.
3 Zimmer, Zachary. Global Ageing in the Twenty-First Century: Challenges, Opportunities and Implications. New York, NY: Routledge, 2016.

4 Christensen K, Doblhammer G, Rau R, Vaupel JW. Ageing populations: the challenges ahead. Lancet, 2009; 374(9696):1196–208.

5 Marengoni A, et al. Coexisting chronic conditions in the older population: variation by health indicators. Eur J Intern Med, 2016; 31:29–34.

6 Blazer D, Wallace R. Cognitive aging: what every geriatric psychiatrist should know. Am J Geriat Psychiatry, 2016; 24(9):776–81.

7 Marengoni A, et al. Aging with multimorbidity: a systematic review of the literature. Ageing Res Ver, 2011; 10:430–9.

8 Todd C, Skelton D. What are the main risk factors for falls among older people and what are the most effective interventions to prevent these falls? Copenhagen, WHO Regional Office for Europe. Health Evidence Network report, 2004.

9 Fried LP, et al. Untangling the concepts of disability, frailty, and comorbidity: implications for improved targeting care. J Gerontol, 2004; 59(3):255–63.

10 Martins AC, Moreira J, Silva C, Silva J, Tonelo C, Baltazar D, Rocha C, Pereira T, Sousa I. Multifactorial screening tool for determining fall risk in community-dwelling adults aged 50 years or over (FallSensing): protocol for a prospective study. JMIR Res Protoc, 2018; 7(8):e10304.

11 Solomon DH. Foreword. In: Osterweil D, Brummel-Smith K, Beck JC. Comprehensive Geriatric Assessment. USA: McGraw Hill, 2000.

12 Devons CA. Comprehensive geriatric assessment: making the most of the aging years. Curr Opin Clin Nutr Metab Care, 2002; 5(1):19–24.

13 Stuck AE, et al. Comprehensive geriatric assessment: a meta-analysis of controlled trials. Lancet, 1993; 342(8878):1032–6.

14 Ward KT, Reuben DB. Comprehensive geriatric assessment. Up-to-Date, 2016; 1–14.

15 Inouye SK, et al. Geriatric syndromes: clinical, research, and policy implications of a core geriatric concept. J Am Geriatr Soc, 2007; 55(5):780–91.

16 Paixão Jr. CM, Reichenhein ME. Uma revisão sobre os instrumentos de avaliação funcional do idoso. Cad Saúde Pública, 2005; 21(1):7–19.

17 Costa EFA. Avaliação Geriátrica Ampla (AGA). In: Liberman A, Freitas EV, Savioli Neto F, Taddei CFG. Diagnóstico e Tratamento em Cardiologia Geriátrica. São Paulo; Editora Manole, 2005.

18 Barnett K, et al. Epidemiology of multimorbidity and implications for health care, research, and medical education: a cross-sectional study. Lancet, 2012; 380(9836):37–43.

19 Ellis G, et al. Comprehensive geriatric assessment for older adults admitted to hospital: meta-analysis of randomised controlled trials. BMJ, 2011; 343:d6553.

20 Baztán JJ, Suárez-García FM, López-Arrieta J, Rodríguez-Mañas L, Rodríguez-Artalejo F. Effectiveness of acute geriatric units on functional decline, living at home, and case fatality among older patients admitted to hospital for acute medical disorders: meta-analysis. BMJ, 2009; 338:b50.

21 Ellis G, Langhorne P. Comprehensive geriatric assessment for older hospital patients. Br Med Bull, 2005; 71:45–59.

22 Wieland D, Hirth V. Comprehensive geriatric assessment. Cancer Control, 2003; 10(6):454–62.

23 Costa EFA, Monego ET. Avaliação Geriátrica Ampla. Revista UFG, 2003; 5(2): 11–15.

24 Guralnik JM et al. Disability as a public health outcome in the aging population. Annu Rev Public Health, 1996; 17:25–46.

25 Ong T. Ageing positively. J Prim Health Care, 2016; 8:86.

26 Kogan AC, Wilber K, Mosqueda L. Person-centered care for older adults with chronic conditions and functional impairment: a systematic literature review. J Am Geriatr Soc, 2016; 64(1):e1–7.

27 Giacalone D, et al. Health and quality of life in an aging population – food and beyond. Food Qual Prefer, 2016; 47:166–70.

28 Duzel E, van Praag H, Sendtner M. Can physical exercise in old age improve memory and hippocampal function? Brain, 2016; 139(Pt 3): 662–73.

29 Mrazek D, et al. Pushing the limits: cognitive, affective, and neural plasticity revealed by an intensive multifaceted intervention. Front Hum Neurosci, 2016; 10:117.

30 Barton J, et al., eds. Green Exercise: Linking Nature, Health and Well-being. New York, NY: Routledge, 2016.

31 Lavallière M, et al. Tackling the challenges of an aging workforce with the use of wearable technologies and the quantified-self. J Facult Minas, 2016; 83(197):38–43.

32 Elsawy B, Higgins KE. The geriatric assessment. Am Fam Physician, 2011; 83(1):48–56.

2 Promoting functional ability and falls prevention

Strategies for healthy aging

Anabela Correia Martins, Daniela Guia,
and Marina Saraiva

Introduction

Healthy aging is the process of optimizing opportunities for physical, social, and mental health to enable older people to take an active part in society without discrimination and to enjoy an independent and good quality of life.[1]

The World Health Organization (WHO) has accepted that this process aims to increase and maintain an individual's participation in activities to improve their quality of life.[2] On the other hand, participation is the involvement of a person in a real-life situation and represents the social perspective of functioning.[3]

Recently, in the Global Strategy and Action Plan for Ageing and Health,[4] the large concept of healthy aging was assumed to be significant for everyone and defined as the process of development and maintenance of functional ability that enables social participation and lifelong well-being.

According to the same document, social participation is determined by individual's intrinsic capacities, such as the combination of all of an individual's physical and mental abilities, environmental factors, and the interaction between both.

The environmental factors, products, and technologies; relationships with friends, family, and caregivers; cultural and social attitudes and values; policy; policies, systems, and services related to transportation, housing, social protection, streets, and parks; social facilities; and health and long-term health care may manifest as barriers or act as facilitators of human functioning.[4]

The Mobility-related Activity and Participation Profile (PAPM) scale allows one to evaluate the difficulties that an individual has in his natural context in carrying out the activities of daily living, namely activities related to social interactions and relationships,

DOI: 10.4324/9781003215271-2

education, employment, money management, and community and social life. It therefore assesses each person's performance in a daily context and in relation to daily activities, that is, the social participation profile. The scale consists of 18 items, rated from 0 to 4, where 0 represents "no difficulty," 1 "slight difficulty," 2 "moderate difficulty," 3 "severe difficulty," 4 "complete difficulty," NA "does not apply." The total score is obtained through the quotient between the sum of the score obtained in each item answered and the number of items answered (0–4). According to the International Classification qualifiers of Functioning, Disability and Health (ICF),[3] a higher score suggests a worse social participation profile.[5]

Falls, defined by the WHO as unexpected and unintentional events in which the individual comes to rest inadvertently on the ground, floor or another lower level, increase the likelihood of loss of autonomy, independence and quality of life in older adults.[6,7] It is estimated that about 30% of individuals older than 65 years suffer at least one fall per year, and that the risk increases to 50% beyond 80 years.[8,9] The potential relationship between functional ability, history of fall and its circumstances, and social participation justifies the growing need for research in this field, to meet the Global Strategy and Plan of Action for Ageing and Health.[4] Indeed, falls represent one of the most critical public issues among older adults.[10]

Despite the fact that falls in the older adult cannot be fully prevented even with the best organized preventive measures, their number may however be significantly reduced through educational strategies raising awareness of the consequences of falls, and with multifactorial and adjusted interventions directed to the risk factors identified at the individual level. An exercise component, including strength, balance, and gait exercises, should always be included in this type of intervention.[11–13]

Reducing fall risk in older individuals is therefore an important public health objective. An important point is to know the functional profile of the older adult population, their motivations and contexts, and signaling individuals at risk of falling, enabling them to develop personalized preventive programs.

Exercise is a fundamental intervention tool in improving the functional ability and quality of life of the person throughout life.[14] There is strong scientific evidence supporting the efficacy of exercise in the prevention of falls in older adults since strength and balance are often compromised in this age group and, consequently, the risk of falls increases.[13] The recommended exercise programs for older adults include aerobic, strengthening, and balancing exercises with the main objective of promoting functional ability and preventing/controlling chronic diseases[15] and falls.

Functional assessment and fall risk screening

To develop an active aging and health promotion program, it is crucial to focus intervention on the person, their needs, and expectations. An individualized and global evaluation is essential, including functional ability, using valid and reliable measuring instruments. Recent studies demonstrated a strong association between history of fall, fear of fall and sedentary behaviors, and functional decline among older adults.[16–18]

Falls are considered the strongest single predictor for future falls and can influence the fear of fall and thus contribute to a loss of independence and disability through the restriction of activities.[19] Fear of fall has been recognized as a potentially debilitating consequence of functional decline, and 30% of the older adult population reported this fear.[20] It may lead to staying home or other self-restriction of activities with debilitating physical and psychological consequences. In addition, it contributes to a sedentary lifestyle, which has implications for functional ability (strength, mobility, gait, balance, and endurance), that is associated with age and risk of falling[20,21] and may also be related to increased mortality in the older adults.[22,23]

Sedentary behavior refers to activities that do not increase energy expenditure substantially above the resting level and includes activities such as sleeping, sitting, lying down, watching television, and other forms of screen-based entertainment.[24]

According to Martínez-Gómez et al., individuals who spent less than 8 hours per day seated had 0.70 times lower risk of mortality compared to individuals with sedentary behavior.[25] The adoption of a healthy and active lifestyle may thus substantially reduce the risk of mortality in older adults.

Functioning can be improved by several factors, either alone or combined, among which exercise and physical activity play a decisive role, and should therefore be integrated into programs for promoting healthy aging. Appropriate measures and screening tools should be envisioned to characterize the functional profile and risk of falling of the older adult. Several functional tests have been validated as reliable measures to assess functional ability and the risk of falling, and to confirm the effect of an intervention plan.[26] The handgrip strength test may help identify patients at increased risk of health deterioration, because handgrip strength is a powerful indicator of overall muscle strength[27] and is associated with lower limb strength.[28] It can predict mortality associated with chronic disease or muscle impairment.[27] This measure can be used to diagnose sarcopenia and frailty in older adults,[29] and to assess muscle strength.[30] Handgrip strength is usually obtained with a handgrip dynamometer. There is no consensus in the literature regarding the position to assess handgrip strength,[29] which may be performed with the individual sitting comfortably and with the dominant arm close to the body (without support), with the shoulder in adduction, the elbow flexed at 90°, the forearm in neutral position.[31,32] During the test, the subject is instructed and encouraged to exert maximum force for 5 seconds.[18] A reduced handgrip strength was associated with a higher risk of falls in the previous 12 months in a previous study.[33] Values below 15 kg and 21 kg in women and men, respectively, indicate fragility and increased risk of falling.[34]

Decreased muscle strength due to the aging process is also related to the risk of falls during gait. Considering the importance of gait for functioning, independence, and mobility,[35,36] it is fundamental to evaluate muscle strength and to prescribe intervention programs aimed at improving strength, particularly in the knee flexor muscles, so as to improve walking performance and to prevent falls.[17]

The 30 Seconds Sit to Stand test is an instrument to evaluate the functional strength of the lower limbs and was shown to be an effective and valid test for the older population residing in the community. It consists of a sit and stand up from a chair, with arms crossed over the chest, as many times as possible for 30 seconds.[18,37] The normative levels for the number of stands depend on age and gender.[38] Changes throughout the aging process, namely the reduction of physical activity levels, decreased gait speed, and muscle strength, are associated with an early or faster decline in mobility.[39,40]

The incidence and prevalence of gait impairment are high in adults living in the community, increasing the risk of falls, institutionalization, and mortality.[41] Several studies used the Timed Up and Go (TUG) test to assess mobility, balance, and risk of fall.[42] This test quantifies functional mobility in seconds.[43] The individual is instructed to sit on a chair (height between 44 and 47 cm)[35] with his back well against its back,[36] being asked to perform the task of getting up from the chair, walk 3 meters as fast as possible, turn and return toward the chair, and sit down again.[43,44,45] The test is performed only once.[46] A score of >10 seconds is indicative of a greater risk of falls.[18,47]

Balance is also essential to carry out activities of daily living. The impairment of this ability increases the likelihood of falls and consequent injuries throughout the lifespan, and could be due to sensorimotor changes, decrease or loss of proprioception, muscular strength, reaction time, visual and vestibular ability, or other pathological conditions.[48] Mobility inherently depends on balance and therefore balance is often assessed through mobility tests including balance, gait, and transfers.[48] The Step test is designed to assess the dynamic standing balance.[49,50] The individual has to go up and down a step (7.5 cm height, 55 cm width, 35 cm depth) as many times as possible, for 15 seconds, always with the same foot. The test is interrupted if loss of balance occurs and the result is given as the number of repetitions performed during the 15 seconds.[50–52] A performance of <10 steps indicates a higher risk of falling.[53] The static balance is evaluated through the 4 Stage Balance Test "Modified."[18] It consists in performing four different feet positions, with progressively increasing degree of difficulty. The individual, with his arms along the body, barefoot and without support, has to hold each position for 10 seconds and only moves to the next position if there is no imbalance during that time.[54,55] The positions that constitute the test are: feet together side by side, semi-tandem, tandem, and one legged stance.[55] Each position is held with eyes open and closed, with the exception of the last position (one-legged stance) that is performed with eyes open. The sequence will be side-by-side stance (eyes open); side-by-side stance (eyes closed); semi-tandem (eyes open), semi-tandem (eyes closed); tandem (eyes open); tandem (eyes closed), and one leg stance (eyes open). The number of positions performed successfully is accounted for.[18] The inability to complete 10 seconds in the tandem stance position with eyes open has been associated with a higher risk of falling and mobility dysfunction.[56,57]

Self-efficacy for exercise and programs for the prevention of falls

Successful programs require individuals to adhere to proposed exercise plans, but there are several factors that may act as barriers to adherence, namely the lack of interest, fear of falling, poor health, low expectations of results, lack of motivation, perceived fragility, or low self-efficacy.[58] Self-efficacy is receiving increasing recognition as a predictor of health behavior change and maintenance.[59] This concept refers to a person's sense of confidence in his or her ability to perform a particular behavior in a variety of circumstances.[59,60] According to Bandura, an individual's persistence and efforts toward specific behavior are closely related to his or her level of self-efficacy.[61–63] Moreover, self-efficacy beliefs contribute to motivation in several ways: they determine the type of activities chosen, the effort to be expended, and the degree of persistence in the effort.[61-63] Therefore, people who have a strong belief in their capabilities to perform an action are more likely to initiate and persist in the given activity and usually have better performance.[60,61,63-65] The self-efficacy theory bases its concept of behavior change on two central points: self-efficacy and outcome expectations. The underlying assumption of social cognitive theory suggests that behavioral change and the maintenance of that behavior are a function of the expectations about one's ability to perform a certain behavior (self-efficacy) and the expectations about the outcome resulting from performing that behavior (outcome expectations).[60,61] Both self-efficacy and outcome expectations play a role in the adoption of health behaviors, the modification of unhealthy habits, and the maintenance of change.[66] Individuals with higher self-efficacy expectations maintain a greater sense of energy during exercise, perceive less effort being expended during exercise, report a more positive effect, and feel more revitalized during and after exercise. In contrast, perceived high physiological strain may weaken one's belief in being able to carry out the activity.[60] Attention should be given to increasing confidence in the older adults to overcome barriers to exercise and achieve relevant fitness outcomes in exercise programs. The level of self-efficacy may promote or limit the motivation to act, meaning that a person will neither be involved in an activity (physical exercise in this case) nor adopt goals with that purpose, unless the person believes he/she is capable of successfully performing it.[67] Therefore, high self-efficacies should be related to better health andfunctioning.[68] Self-efficacy assessment is thus a fundamental tool in the prescription of an exercise plan, as this dimension strongly determines individual adherence to the program. The self-efficacy beliefs will contribute to the success of these intervention plans. People who have a high self-efficacy can experience scenarios of success while those who rate themselves as ineffective are more likely to experience scenarios of failure undermining their adherence to the prescribed plan.[68,69]

Self-efficacy can be assessed through the Self-efficacy for Exercise Scale, originally developed by Schwarzer and Renner, in 2009.[70] This instrument assesses the confidence that the individual has in his/her ability to perform exercise. It is a 5-item scale that analyzes the confidence an individual presents to perform physical exercise according to different emotional states, such as feeling worried and troubled, feeling depressed, feeling tense, feeling tired, and feeling busy. The questionnaire is administered by interview, each of these items is graded through a 4-point Likert scale, 1 being defined as "not at all true," 2 "slightly true," 3 "moderately true," and 4 "completely true." The total score results from the sum of the scores of each item, varying between 5 and 20. The higher the score, the greater the confidence or the sense of self-efficacy for exercise.[71]

The WHO[3] indicates that environmental factors constitute the "physical, social and attitudinal environment in which people live and lead their lives." There are two levels, the first relates to the individual environment nearby, for example, housing, school, and the workplace, and the second refers to a broader social level, such as cultural influences, individual and social attitudes, norms and services, existing systems and policies. Environmental changes, both at home and in the public environment (railings, handrails, non-slip surfaces), improve the living conditions of people in general, and older adults in particular.[72] Assessing the individual's perception of home hazards that may contribute to an increased risk of falling is relevant to the health professional, providing a means to identify the risks and intervene with educational intervention, advising for architectural changes, to minimize risks. The Home Safety Checklist for Fall Prevention is a checklist designed to identify home hazards in each room of a person's home, namely the hallways, stairs, living or dining room, kitchen, bathroom, bedroom, and outdoors.[73,74] It is a 38-item list using a 3-point scale from 0 (indicating "no risk"), 1 (indicating "risk"), and 99 (indicating "does not apply"). A risk score is produced both for each room and for the home in general.[73,74]

Exercise-based intervention programs

Exercise is a fundamental intervention tool in improving the functional ability and quality of life of the person throughout life, and the relevant literature has been supporting the efficacy of exercise for the prevention of falls in older adults.[12]

A systematic review and meta-analysis[75] established strong evidence that exercise interventions reduce the rate and risk of falling in community-dwelling older adults. Furthermore, it suggests programs with more than 3 hours/week of exercise, involving balance, strength, and walking exercises as the more effective for the prevention of falls and to promotefunctioning. Physical activity constitutes a protector factor for falls in persons aged over 60 years. Moreover, physically active older adults are 0.75 times less prone for falling than those who are physically inactive or sedentary.[76]

The Otago Exercise Program (OTAGO) is commonly applied as an intervention to reduce the risk of falling and it incorporates strength exercises of the lower limbs and balance,[77] with moderate intensity exercises, to be performed for about 30 minutes, at least three times a week. Walking on alternate days can be associated, at least twice a week.[78] This program is significantly effective in increasing the muscular strength of the lower limbs, in improving balance and gait and, consequently, in preventing falls in older adults, and can be used daily in clinical practice and/or as an exercise program to be done at home.[79] Recently, a systematic review aimed at identifying modified versions of the OTAGO program, reported improvements on balance and functional ability, in formats that included exercise associated with vestibular or multisensory balance exercises, use of augmented reality, exercises in group with a physiotherapist or with DVD support.[80] However, it remains unclear if these adapted formats are as effective as the original OTAGO program, and which modified format is comparatively more effective, considering that different adaptations of the OTAGO were considered in different studies.[80] However, exercise programs incorporated in technological tools were associated with significant improvements in balance, mobility, and prevention of falls in older adults.[81]

Interventions based on the use of biofeedback provide individuals with additional information about their performance, allowing them to be able to develop changes in their behavior or posture, and consequently, leading to better performance of the tasks. In the literature, evidence exists supporting the integration of visual biofeedback in the balance training programs, providing additional benefits to improve balance when compared to traditional exercise programs or no intervention.[82] Molina et al. identified the benefits of intervention programs incorporating interactive games (Exergames) in the physical function of older adults, and although the data were inconclusive, it was demonstrated that the motivational aspect is reinforced with the combination of technology and exercise.[83] This may be due to the existence of a strong motivational component in this type of intervention, which may also improve adherence to intervention programs for active aging. A home-based, multidimensional exercise program in community-dwelling older adults with functional impairment is feasible and effective in improving functional performance, despite limited supervision. Minimally supervised exercise is safe and can improve functional performance in older adults.[84] Several studies provided support for the use of therapeutic exercise in minimizing loss of stability in the older adult through balance and mobility improvement, hence reducing the risk of falling during the aging process.[42,85] Regarding the technologies adopted in these intervention programs, several studies have also demonstrated a positive impact on users' social participation. However, it is important to guarantee that equipment and associated training are provided by skilled professionals and that users give input in the selection of their assistive device in order to achieve a better performance in everyday tasks, reducing the likelihood of rejection and abandonment and enhancing lifelong independence.[86]

Conclusions

The implementation of global assessment strategies that include functional indicators and using valid and reliable measuring instruments is a major necessity, which could warrant significant contributions for decreasing the risks of falling, loss of independence, and loss of autonomy. Promoting healthy aging by increasing and maintaining an individual's functional ability contributes to enhance his/her participation and well-being throughout life. Thus, it will be possible to design appropriate interventions that meet the needs and expectations of each individual.

Exercise programs, particularly those including strengthening, balance and gait exercises, should be an integral part of the recommended intervention programs for promoting healthy aging, promoting social participation, quality of life, and preventing chronic illness and/or falls. Exercise programs, whether implemented in a more conventional group or individual manner, or using technologies, should be developed and prescribed by qualified professionals.

Key points

- Disability and risk of falling are important factors to take into account during the aging process.
- Early fall risk screening and multifactorial assessment of personal and environmental characteristics are the starting point for prescribing exercise and multifactorial interventions.
- Interventions based on exercise, focused on strengthening and balance programs are effective in preventing falls and promoting healthy aging.
- These training programs should be developed and prescribed by qualified professionals, such as a physical therapist.
- Promotion of self-efficacy for exercise can contribute to increase adherence to the programs.

References

1 European Commission. Healthy Ageing: A Challenge for Europe. Stockholm, Sweden: Swedish National Institute for Public Health. 2007.

2 World Health Organization. Towards a Common Language for Functioning, Disability and Health. Geneva: World Health Organization. 2002.

3 World Health Organization (WHO). International Classification of Functioning, Disability and Health. Geneva: Classification, Assessment, Surveys and Terminology Team. 2001.

4 World Health Organization (WHO). Global Strategy and Action Plan on Ageing and Health. Geneva: World Health Organization. 2017. https://www.who.int/ageing/WHO-GSAP-2017.pdf?ua=1. Acedido em dezembro 18, 2018.

5 Martins AC. Development and initial validation of the Activities and Participation Profile related to Mobility (APPM). BMC Health Serv Res. 2016;16(3):78–79.

6 World Health Organization (WHO). WHO global report on falls prevention in older age. WHO Libr Cat Data. 2007;53: ISBN9789241563536

7 Coutinho EDSF, Silva SD. Uso de medicamentos como fator de risco para fratura grave decorrente de queda em idosos. Cad Saude Publica. 2002;18(5):1359–1366.

8 Gardner MM, Robertson MC, Campbell AJ. Exercise in preventing falls and fall related injuries in older people: a review of randomised controlled trials. Br J Sports Med. 2000;34(1):7–17.

9 Sachetti A, Vidmar MF, Marinho M, Schneider RH, Wibelinger M. Risco de quedas em idosos com osteoporose. Rev Bras Ciências da Saúde. 2010;24(8):22–26.

10 World Health Organization (WHO). Health Literacy: The Solid Facts. Copenhagen, Denmark: WHO. 2013.

11 American Geriatrics Society/British Geriatrics Society (AGS/BGS). Summary of the updated American Geriatrics Society/British Geriatrics Society Clinical Practice Guideline for Prevention of Falls in Older Persons. J Am Geriatr Soc. 2011;59:148–157.

12 National Institute for Health and Care Excellence (NICE). Falls: Assessment and prevention of falls in older people. NICE clinical guideline 161. 2013.

13 Gillespie LD, Robertson MC, Gillespie WJ. Interventions for preventing falls in older people living in the community. Cochrane Database Syst Rev. 2009;2(2):CD007146.

14 Silva TO Da, Freitas RSDF, Monteiro MR, Borges SDM. Avaliação da capacidade física e quedas em idosos ativos e sedentários da comunidade. Rev Bras Clin Médica. 2010;8(5):392–398.

15 Matsudo SM, Keihan V, Matsudo R, Barros L. Atividade física e envelhecimento: aspectos epidemiológicos. Rev Bras Med Esporte. 2001;7(1):2–13.

16 Choi K, Jeon G, Cho S. Prospective study on the impact of fear of falling on functional decline among community dwelling elderly women. Int J Env Res Public Heal. 2017;14(5):469.

17 Cebolla EC, Rodacki ALF, Bento PCB. Balance, gait, functionality and strength: comparison between elderly fallers and non-fallers. Braz J Phys Ther. 2015;19(2):146–151.

18 Martins AC, Moreira J, Silva C, et al. Multifactorial screening tool for determining fall risk in community-dwelling adults aged 50 years or over (FallSensing): protocol for a prospective study. J Med Internet Res. 2018;20(8):1–11.

19 Stel VS, Smit JH, Pluijm SMF, Lips P. Consequences of falling in older men and women and risk factors for health service use and functional decline. Age Ageing. 2004;33(1):58–65.

20 Arfken C, Birge SJ. The prevalence and correlates of fear of falling in elderly persons living. Am J Public Health. 1993;84(4):565–570.

21 Jung D. Fear of falling in older adults: comprehensive review. Asian Nurs Res (Korean Soc Nurs Sci). 2008;2(4):214–222.

22 Wadhwa D, Hande D. Effectiveness of Otago Exercise Program on reducing the fall risk in elderly: single case report. Imp J Interdiscip Res. 2016;2(6):614–618.

23 De Rezende LFM, Rey-López JP, Matsudo VKR, Luiz ODC. Sedentary behavior and health outcomes among older adults: a systematic review. BMC Public Health. 2014;14(333):1–9.

24 Pate RR, Neill JRO, Lobelo F. The evolving definition of "Sedentary". Exerc Sport Sci Rev. 2008;36:173–178.

25 Martínez-Gómez D, Guallar-castillón P, León-muñoz LM, López-garcía E, Rodríguez-artalejo F. Combined impact of traditional and non-traditional health behaviors on mortality: a national prospective cohort study in Spanish older adults. BMC Med. 2013; 11(47):1–10.

26 Amada TY, Emura SD. Effectiveness of sit-to-stand tests for evaluating physical functioning and fall risk in community-dwelling elderly. Hum Perform Meas. 2015;12:1–7.

27 Rantanen T, Volpato S, Ferrucci L, Heikkinen E, Fried LP, Guralnik JM. Handgrip strength and cause-specific and total mortality in older disabled women: exploring the mechanism. J Am Geriat Soc. 2003;51(5):636–641.

28 Aadahl M, Beyer N, Linneberg A, Thuesen BH, Jørgensen T. Grip strength and lower limb extension power in 19-72-year-old Danish men and women: the Health 2006 study. BMJ Open. 2011;1(e00019):1–8.

29 Sousa-Santos AR, Amaral TF. Differences in handgrip strength protocols to identify sarcopenia and frailty – a systematic review. BMC Geriatr. 2017;17(238):1–21.

30 Prata MG, Scheicher ME. Effects of strength and balance training on the mobility, fear of falling and grip strength of elderly female fallers. J Bodyw Mov Ther. 2015;19(4):646–650.

31 Bastiaanse LP, Hilgenkamp TIM, Echteld MA, Evenhuis HM. Prevalence and associated factors of sarcopenia in older adults with intellectual disabilities. Res Dev Disabil. 2012;33(6):2004–2012.

32 Campbell TM, Vallis LA. Predicting fat-free mass index and sarcopenia in assisted-living older adults. Age (Omaha). 2014;36(9674):1–13.

33 Lenardt MH, Carneiro NHK, Betiolli SE, Binotto MA, Ribeiro DK de MN, Teixeira FFR. Factors associated with decreased hand grip strength in the elderly. Esc Anna Nery - Rev Enferm. 2016;20(4):1–7.

34 Lanziotti S, Gomes V, Máximo LS, Marcos J, Dias D, Dias RC. Comparação entre diferentes pontos de corte na classificação do perfil de fragilidade de idosos comunitários. Geriatr Gerontol. 2011;5(3):130–135.

35 Kerrigan DC, Lee LW, Collins JJ, et al. Reduced hip extension during walking: healthy elderly and fallers versus young adults. Arch Phys Med Rehabil. 2001;82(1):26–30.

36 Kwon IS, Oldaker S, Schrager M, Talbot LA, Fozard JL, Metter EJ. Relationship between muscle strength and the time taken to complete a standardized walk-turn-walk test. J Gerontol Biol Sci. 2001;56(9): 398–404.

37 Jones CJ, Rikli RE, Beam WC. A 30-s chair-stand test as a measure of lower body strength in community-residing older adults. Res Q Exerc Sport. 1999;70(2):113–119.

38 Center for Disease Control and Prevention. ASSESSMENT: 30-Second Chair Stand. 2017. https://www.cdc.gov/steadi/pdf/STEADI-Assessment-30Sec-508.pdf. Acedido em 18 de dezembro, 2018.

39 Ho SC, Woo J, Yuen YK, Sham A, Chan SG. Predictors of mobility decline: the Hong Kong old-old study. J Gerontol Med Sci. 1997;52(6):356–362.

40 Buchman AS, Wilson ÃRS, Boyle PA, Tang ÃY, Fleischman DA, Bennett DA. Physical activity and leg strength predict decline in mobility. J Am Geriatr Soc. 2007;55(10):1618–1623.

41 Verghese J, Levalley ÃA, Hall ÃCB, Katz ÃMJ. Epidemiology of gait disorders in community-residing older adults. J Am Geriatr Soc. 2006;54(2):255–261.

42 Cadore EL, Rodríguez-Mañas L, Sinclair A, Izquierdo M. Effects of different exercise interventions on risk of falls, gait ability, and balance in physically frail older adults: a systematic review. Rejuvenation Res. 2013;16(2):105–114.

43 Podsiadlo D, Richardson S. The timed "Up & Go": a test of basic functional mobility for frail elderly persons. J Am Geriatr Soc. 1991;39(2):142–148.

44 Siggeirsdóttir K, Jónsson BY, Jónsson H, Iwarsson S. The timed 'Up & Go' is dependent on chair type. Clin Rehabil. 2002;16(6):609–616.

45 Beauchet O, Fantino B, Allali G, Muir S, Montero-Odasso M, Annweiler C. Timed Up and Go test and risk of falls in older adults: a systematic review. J Nutr Health Aging. 2011;15(10):933–938.

46 Rehabilitation Measures Database. https://www.sralab.org/rehabilitation-measures/hand-held-dynamometergrip-strength. Acedido em fevereiro 22, 2018.

47 Rose DJ, Jones CJ, Lucchese N. Predicting the probability of falls in community-residing older adults using the 8-foot up-and-go: a new measure of functional mobility. J Aging Phys Act. 2002;10(4):466–475.

48 L. Sturnieks D, St George R, R. Lord S. Balance disorders in the elderly. Neurophysiol Clin Neurophysiol. 2008;38(6):467–478.

49 Mercer V, Freburger J, Chang S, Purser J. Step test scores are related to measures of activity and participation in the first 6 months after stroke. Phys Ther. 2009;89(10):1061–1071.

50 Hill KD, Bernhardt J, McGann AM, Maltese D, Berkovits D. A new test of dynamic standing balance for stroke patients: reliability, validity and comparison with healthy elderly. Physiother Can. 1996;48(4):257–262.

51 Grimmer-Somers K, Hillier S, Young A, Sutton M, Lizarondo L. CAHE Neurological Outcomes Calculator User Manual: Monitoring Patient Status Over Time Using Common Neurological Outcome Measures. Adelaide, SA: University of South Australia - Centre for Allied Health Evidence. 2009.

52 Isles R, Choy N, Steer M, Nitz J. Normal values of balance tests in women aged 20–80. J Am Geriatr Soc. 2004;52(8):1367–1372.

53 Martins A, Silva J, Santos A, Madureira J, Alcobia J, Ferreira L, et al. Case-based study of metrics derived from instrumented fall risk assessment tests. Preprints. 2016;2016080132:1–12.

54 Rossiter-Fornoff JE, Wolf SL, Wolfson LI, Buchner DM. A cross-sectional validation study of the FICSIT common data base static balance measures. Frailty and Injuries: Cooperative Studies of Intervention Techniques. J Gerontol A Biol Sci Med Sci. 1995;50(6): M291–M297.

55 Thomas JC, Odonkor C, Griffith L, Holt N, Percac-Lima S, Leveille S, et al. Reconceptualizing balance: attributes associated with balance performance. Exp Gerontol. 2014;57:218–223.

56 Murphy MA, Olson SL, Protas EJ, Overby AR. Screening for falls in community-dwelling elderly. J Aging Phys Act. 2003;11(1):66–80.

57 Shubert TE, Schrodt LA, Mercer VS, Busby-Whitehead J, Giuliani CA. Are scores on balance screening tests associated with mobility in older adults? J Geriatr Phys Ther. 2006;29(1):35–39.

58 Peel N, Bell RAR, Smith K. Queensland Stay On Your Feet® Community Good Practice Guidelines – Preventing Falls, Harm From Falls and Promoting Healthy Active Ageing in Older Queenslanders. Brisbane: Queensland Health. 2008.

59 Strecher VJ, Devellis BM, Becker MH, Rosenstock IM. The role of self-efficacy in achieving health behavior change. Spring. 1986;13(1):73–91.

60 Lee LL, Arthur A, Avis M. Using self-efficacy theory to develop interventions that help older people overcome psychological barriers to physical activity: a discussion paper. Int J Nurs Stud. 2008;45(11): 1690–1699.

61 Bandura A. Self-efficacy: toward a unifying of behavioral change theory. Psychol Rev. 1978;84:139–161.

62 Bandura A. Perceived self-efficacy in the exercise of personal agency. Rev Española Pedagog. 1990;48(187):397–427.

63 Bandura A. Social cognitive theory: an agentic perspective. Annu Rev Psychol. 2001;52(1):1–26.

64 Buckelew SP, Huyser B, Hewett JE, Johnson JC, Conway R, Parker JC, Kay DR. Self-efficacy predicting outcome among fibromyalgia subjects. Arthritis & Rheum. 1996;9:97–104.

65 Schwarzer R, Renner B. Social-cognitive predictors of health behavior: action self-efficacy and coping self-efficacy. Health Psychol. 2000;19(5): 487–495.

66 Brassington GS, Atienza A, Perczek RE, DiLorenzo TM, King AC. Intervention-related cognitive versus social mediators of exercise adherence in the elderly. Am J Prevent Med. 2002;23(2, Suppl 1):80–86.

67 Ponton MK, Edmister JH, Ukeiley LS, Seiner JM. Understanding the role of self-efficacy in engineering education. J Eng Educ. 2001;90(2):247–251.

68 Martins A. Programas de Exercício e Prevenção de Quedas: Um estudo piloto para identificar necessidades dos idosos a residir na comunidade. In: Revista Ibero-americana Gerontologia. Coimbra: Associação Nacional de Gerontologia Social. 2013:27–46.

69 Bandura A. Human agency in social cognitive theory. Am Psychol. 1989;44:1175–1184.

70 Schwarzer R, Renner B. Health-Specific Self-Efficacy Scales. 2009. https://userpage.fu-berlin.de/health/healself.pdf. Acedido em 18 de dezembro, 2018.

71 Martins AC, Silva C, Moreira J, Rocha C, Gonçalves A. Escala de autoeficácia para o exercício: validação para a população portuguesa. In: Pocinho R, Ferreira SM, Anjos VN. (coord.). Conversas de Psicologia e do Envelhecimento Ativo. 1a Edição. Coimbra: Associação Portuguesa Conversas de Psicologia; 2017:126–141.

72 European Public Health Association (EUPHA). Falls among older adults in the EU-28: Key facts from the available statistics. 2015. http://tinyurl.com/gqzhfje. Acedido em 15 de abril, 2016.

73 Center for Disease Control and Prevention (CDC). Check for Safety, A Home Fall Prevention Checklist for Older Adults. Prevention. 2015. https://www.cdc.gov/steadi/pdf/check_for_safety_brochure-a.pdf. Acedido em 18 de dezembro, 2018.

74 Silva C, Andrade I, Martins AC. Preventing Falls – I Can Do It. Saarbrucken, Germany: Scholar's Press. 2015.

75 Sherrington C, Michaleff ZA, Fairhall N, et al. Exercise to prevent falls in older adults: an updated systematic review and meta-analysis. Br J Sport Med. 2017;51:1749–1757.

76 Thibaud M, Bloch F, Tournoux-facon C, et al. Impact of physical activity and sedentary behaviour on fall risks in older people: a systematic review and meta-analysis of observational studies. Eur Rev Aging Phys Act. 2012;9(5):5–15.

77 Bjerk M, Brovold T, Skelton DA, Bergland A. A falls prevention programme to improve quality of life, physical function and falls efficacy in older people receiving home help services: study protocol for a randomised controlled trial. BMC Health Serv Res. 2017;17(1):1–9.

78 Accident Compensation Corporation (ACC). Otago Exercise Programme to Prevent Falls in Older Adults: A Home-based, Individually Tailored Strength and Balance Retraining Programme. New Zealand: University of Otago. 2007.

79 Patel NN. The effects of Otago Exercise Programme for fall prevention in elderly people. Int J Physiother. 2015;2(4):633–639.

80 Martins AC, Santos C, Silva C, Baltazar D, Moreira J, Tavares N. Does modified Otago Exercise Program improves balance in older people? A systematic review. Prev Med Rep. 2018;11:231–239.

81 Duque G, Boersma D, Loza-Diaz G, Hassan S, Suarez H, Geisinger D et al. Effects of balance training using a virtual-reality system in older fallers. Clin Interv Aging. 2013;8:257–263.

82 Alhasan H, Hood V, Mainwaring F. The effect of visual biofeedback on balance in elderly population: a systematic review. Clin Interv Aging. 2017;12:487–497.

83 Molina KI, Ricci NA, Moraes SA De, Perracini MR. Virtual reality using games for improving physical functioning in older adults: a systematic review. J Neuroeng Rehabil. 2014;11(1):1–20.

84 Nelson ME, Layne JE, Bernstein MJ, et al. The effects of multidimensional home-based exercise on functional performance in elderly people. J Gerontol Ser A Biol Sci Med Sci. 2004;59(2):M154–M160.

85 Kulkarni N, Pouliasi K. Impact of group exercise programme on fall risk in elderly individuals: a pilot study. Int J Heal Sci Res. 2017;7(4):265–274.

86 Martins A, Pinheiro J, Farias B, Jutai J. Psychosocial impact of assistive technologies for mobility and their implications for active ageing. Technologies. 2016;4(3):28.

3 Physical exercise applied to older people

Inês Cipriano and Telmo Pereira

Introduction

Being old is a challenge. Growing old with quality implies effort and dedication throughout life. Aging is a natural and physiological process whose effects vary from person to person, but it is within everyone's reach to slow its evolution and promote successful aging. Contrary to popular belief, its process is not unalterable, as most of the changes that occur in the older adult are due to extrinsic factors.[1] Since aging is a global phenomenon, across all and in all countries, it is also a triumph of modern society in that it is directly related to the improvement of health care. In Portugal in 2017, over 21.5% of the resident population was over 65, of these, 13.8% were over 85 years. These are revealing data from an aging population,[2] challenging the need to adapt health care to the existing population. Serra and Silva[3] stress that the costs associated with health care increase in direct proportion to aging, being more concentrated in the last two years of life, regardless of age, so people have started living longer, making it important to ensure that these years of life are lived to the highest quality, always taking into account the sustainability of care.

It is important to emphasize the idea already presented by several scholars,[4] by pointing out that regardless of the health care available, each individual has responsibility for the success of their own aging, since it is within human nature to set goals and achieve them. To this end, it is relevant that each person has knowledge about the naturalness of the aging process, develops a critical awareness of it, and suits their life goals. Given the above, and considering the various areas of health care available, we highlight the opinion of Dias et al.[5] who report that physical activity, performed on a regular basis, allows healthy aging, with an impact on improving the quality of life of the older adult, thus "giving more life to the years and not just more years to life."

DOI: 10.4324/9781003215271-3

Based on the above, this chapter aims to explain the framework of exercise in promoting healthy aging, highlighting aspects such as aging, the prescription of exercise in geriatrics and gerontology, the benefits of regular practice, and what are the biggest challenges for the successful implementation of these programs.

Aging: physiological changes

From the point of view of the professional who implements a physical exercise program, it is important to have sound knowledge about the aging process, namely in terms of body composition, cardiorespiratory capacity, the musculoskeletal system, central nervous system, and sensory and perceptual system, among others.

Body composition

Body composition assessment (studied through auxology and kinanthropometry) is an important component in multidimensional functional assessment, particularly in individuals over 65 years of age,[6] being a tool for surveillance and preventive intervention. The concept of body composition of the organism can be made according to several models, starting from a unicompartmental approach, which corresponds to a single weight. There is also the bicompartmental model, which corresponds to the weight divided into fat mass and lean mass, and the multicompartmental model, where the subdivision of lean mass into its constituents is performed.[7,8] Thus, the fat mass corresponds to the total body fat, and is mainly composed of mobilizable fat, consisting mainly of triglycerides and located in the subcutaneous, peri-visceral, and muscular regions, and also the essential fat in the peri-neural, intramedullary region and cell membranes. Lean mass corresponds to body weight without fat, consisting mainly of muscle tissue, connective tissue, and visceral mass. Normal values vary according to age and gender, and an increase in fat mass and its distribution is expected with advancing age, with a decrease in the peripheral region and an increase in the abdominal region. A decrease in lean mass is also expected due to the decrease in total water: decrease in cell mass, predominance of muscle and mostly bone minerals.[9] Spirduso et al.[10] stated that body weight stabilizes in the fifth decade and tends to decrease in the seventh decade, but fat mass may continue to increase.

Cardiorespiratory capacity

Regarding lung volumes, there is an increase in lung compliance, which, together with a reduction in respiratory muscle strength and a decrease in thoracic mobility (kyphosis, calcification), causes a decrease in vital capacity. Functional Residual Capacity (CRF) corresponds to the air volume in the lungs at the end of exhalation, and the Residual Volume (VR) is the volume of gas that remains in the lungs after forced expiration, and both increase with age. Other parameters that change with age are Forced Vital Capacity (FVC) and Forced Expiratory Volume in 1 second (FEV_1), both decreasing with aging, as well as their relationship, which corresponds to the Tiffeneau Index (IT). From the cardiac point of view, the most noticeable changes are the reduction in cardiac output and maximum heart rate, increased blood pressure, and peripheral vascular resistance, which are associated with decreased oxygen consumption. All of these factors associated with other variables may contribute to a decreased ability to perform muscle work, such as decreased frequency and range of ventilatory movements as well as expired air volume.[11] Decline in cardiovascular fitness is mainly due to changes in body composition and respiratory function associated with decreased levels of physical activity in aging.

Musculoskeletal system

Aging is also associated with significant muscular changes, and the existing literature emphasizes that muscle parameters, such as fiber size, number, and diameter, as well as amplitude and velocity, show significant decreases in inverse proportionality to the use of muscle segments.[10,12]

Correia and Silva[11] list two main factors for decreased strength in the older adult: the first, the loss of muscle mass due to atrophy and decrease in the number of muscle fibers; and the second factor is changes in the metabolism of contractile proteins.

Decreased strength plays a role in lower limb strength rather than upper limb, and is often associated with a significant increase in the risk of falling. Atrophy occurs mainly in the large muscle groups of the thigh region, which, according to the aforementioned authors, presents a greater decline in the capacity to produce maximum strength, representing an increase in the difficulty in performing daily life tasks.[11] Ascension et al.[13] also point out the drastic reduction in force at higher speeds, resulting not only from the decreased ability to produce maximum force but also from a slower motor response to contraction and relaxation.

The aging process is also a consequence of less use of different muscle groups, reducing their stimulation, power, speed, flexibility, and precision of movement.[14]

Central nervous system

The central nervous system is widely studied in geriatrics and gerontology, as it is strongly affected by aging, namely in terms of cellular functioning, and the reduction of neurons, leading to the reduction of fibers and nerve bundles, reducing the ability to transmit and receive nerve impulses, resulting in decreased synapses.[15] Weight loss and decreased brain volume, increased connective tissue, hypoxemia, and progressive increase in cerebral vascular resistance are physiological changes that induce changes in the ability to perform simple tasks.[16]

Sensory and perceptual system

Increased senescence contributes to hearing loss, decreased visual acuity, and changes in proprioception. Older people's hearing decreases through various degenerative processes, including cochlea (presbycusis), eardrum thickening, reduced earwax production, increased middle ear ossicle stiffness (otosclerosis), and auditory nerve atrophy.[17] Hearing loss becomes more evident from the fifth decade of life and worsens with aging, making it difficult to distinguish between the sounds of the voice and the environment, and hindering communication, consequently leading to isolation and compromising the ability of interaction with the environment.

Vision is especially sensitive to the effect of age, with visual aging essentially translated by problems in the perception of distant objects, depth, and sensitivity to obfuscation.[18] In the interaction developed with older people, the changes mentioned above are frequently observed, which may manifest as the difficulty in integrating activities such as walking on uneven or stepped floors, group activities with throwing objects, and distance assessment in the execution of exercises.

Proprioception, or kinesthesia, corresponds to the transmission and processing of information by the nervous system.[19] Thus, older people have greater difficulty in performing movements, and this decrease in the ability to properly recognize segmental position, associated with reduced sensitivity, can cause problems in postural control, with increased difficulty in gait control and an increase in the time required to correct gait in the face of obstacles and/or unforeseen variations. One way to minimize this difficulty is to walk slowly to avoid accidents such as falls.

Physical exercise prescription

Levels of physical exercise

According to the World Health Organization, physical exercise is defined as any body movement produced by the energy-consuming skeletal muscles, thus comprising all conscious practice of physical activity, performed for a specific purpose and well-delineated in time, with or without prescription and is generally a planned practice.[20]

The intensity applied to the exercises can be measured absolutely or relatively: the absolute intensity corresponds to the amount of energy used by the body per minute of activity, measured as metabolic equivalent or MET[1]; relative intensity corresponds to the level of effort required, being scored on a scale of 0–10, where 0 corresponds to the state of rest and 10 the maximum effort. Thus, exercises are prescribed using various levels of intensity:

- Light intensity: <3 METs – corresponds to walking, housework, stretching;
- Moderate Intensity: 3–5.9 METs – there is an increase in respiratory and heart rate, and the individual is able to speak but not to sing. Corresponds to water activities, brisk walking or gardening;
- Vigorous Intensity: >6 METs – One can no longer speak more than a few words without stopping. It corresponds to activities such as jogging, aerobics and intense gardening.

Spirduso et al.[10] also proposed an additional classification by function levels:

- Physically dependent: A person who cannot perform some basic tasks of daily life, including dressing, bathing, eating, and walking. These people are dependent on others for basic life needs.
- Physically fragile: People who can perform the basic tasks of life, but cannot perform all the tasks necessary to be independent.
- Physically independent: Independent people, usually without symptoms of chronic illness. However, many with health changes

that can be aggravated leading to a state of "physically fragile" in the event of any injury or worsening of symptoms.

- Physically fit: People who exercise at least twice a week, and who are committed to improving their health. They have a low risk of diminishing their function.
- Physically remarkable: People who train daily, who compete, or are committed to practicing sports in a recreational way.

Physical exercise recommendations

Older adult without chronic disease

In 2011, the World Health Organization published recommendations for physical exercise in people over 65 to improve cardiorespiratory and muscular function, decrease cardiovascular risk factors, and decrease cognitive decline and depression.[21,22] These recommendations suggest: (1) the practice of more than 150 minutes of moderate intensity aerobic exercise every day of the week; (2) more than 75 minutes of vigorous aerobic exercise every day of the week; and (3) the combination of both possibilities described in (1) and (2). To maximize benefits, it proposes an increase in the duration of the straining sessions up to 300 minutes per week at moderate to vigorous intensity.

In people with greater mobility limitations but at risk of falling, the World Health Organization suggests performing exercises for the largest muscle groups two or more times a week.[22] For sedentary older people, it is recommended to start with small efforts, with a progressive increase in the intensity and duration of the exercise.

The American College of Sports Medicine has used the FITT[2] principle, developing an exercise prescription plan for the older adult, with a set of recommendations, which we describe below.[23,24] For cardiorespiratory training, a frequency of 5 or more days per week of moderate intensity activity, or 3 days per week of vigorous intensity is proposed. This should be measured on a scale ranging from 0 to 10, with 5–6 intensity being moderate and 7–8 intensity being vigorous. A suitable instrument for this intensity assessment is Borg's Perceived Effort Scale.[25] Practice time should consist of 10-minute series, up to a total of 150/300 minutes per week, or 20–30 (60 minutes for biggest benefit) minutes a day.

The typology of training should not cause orthopedic stress; hence, the practice of exercise bike, water activities, and walking for less effort-tolerant people should be warranted. Regarding strength training, the American College of Sports Medicine suggests a frequency of two times or more per week, of moderate (60–70% of 1RM[3]) or mild (40–50% of 1RM) intensity. If 1RM is not measured, the intensity should be moderate to vigorous on a scale of 0–10.

For flexibility training, a frequency of two times or more per week is proposed. In this plane, the intensity is evaluated by the muscular extension, corresponding to the intended intensity to the point where a slight discomfort is triggered. The exercise time corresponds to maintaining the slight discomfort position for 30–60 seconds. The exercises should preferably be static avoiding fast movements. As final recommendations, the American College of Sports Medicine emphasizes the importance of training to seek progression that is favorable to the practice and enhances the evolution of an individual's aerobic capacity in the early stages of exercise training.[23,24]

Older adult with chronic disease

For the prescription of exercise in the older adult with chronic diseases, the recommendations provided by Zaleski et al.[26] constitute an important contribution to the adapted prescription of physical exercise, which is presented in an adapted version in Table 3.1.

Best exercise

Taking into account the recommendations of the World Health Organization[22] and the American College of Sports Medicine,[23,24] the types of exercise vary according to the prior assessment of the older person's health conditions, allowing for an exercise prescription adjusted to interests, needs, and resources available for continued physical activity aimed at improving overall quality of life. Thus, some of the exercises most often used for the older adult are those involving large muscle groups, aerobic workouts, especially lower limb strength training, and balance to prevent the risk of falls, and improve flexibility and endurance.

Older old physical fitness rating scale

Rikli and Jones[27,28] proposed a test battery, called Functional Fitness Test, to assess the functional fitness of the older adult. The authors defined physical fitness as being an ability to perform the tasks of daily living safely and without signs of extreme fatigue. This test battery consists of a set of exercises that allow for the evaluation

Table 3.1 Schema for the prescription of exercise in the older adult with chronic diseases

ACSM FITT	Hypertension	Diabetes mellitus II	Dyslipidemia
Frequency	7× week	3–7 day/week	>5 day/week
Intensity	Moderate	Moderate to vigorous	Moderate
Time	30–60 min/day	10–30 min/day to make up the total of 150 min/week	30–60 min/day with best weight loss benefits (50–60 min/day)
Type	Aerobic	Aerobic	Aerobic
Complement 1	Muscle strength training >2 days/week (not consecutive). Moderate to vigorous intensity; 8–10 exercises; >1 set of 8–12 repetitions.	Muscle strength training >2 days/week (not consecutive). Moderate to vigorous intensity; 8–10 exercises; >1 set of 10–15 repetitions.	Muscle strength training >2 days/week (not consecutive). Moderate to vigorous intensity; 8–10 exercises; >1 set of 10–15 repetitions.
Complement 2	Flexibility training >2 days/week at least 10 min/day.	Flexibility training >2 days/week at least 10 min/day.	Flexibility training >2 days/week at least 10 min/day.
Complement 3	Balance training if there is a risk of falling.	Balance training if there is a risk of falling.	Balance training if there is a risk of falling.
Special considerations	Encourage patients to exercise in the morning for immediate benefits in blood pressure during the day.	The combination of aerobic and endurance training helps to balance blood glucose levels more effectively than individualized training. Avoid inactivity two consecutive days. Vigorous intensity allows higher calorie expenditure, which are objective in progression.	The objective should be to perform exercises of large muscle groups that maximize energy expenditure.

ACSM – American College of Sports Medicine.
Source: Adapted from Zaleski et al.[26]

of physiological capabilities, such as flexibility, aerobic endurance, speed, agility, dynamic balance, as well as anthropometric indicators of interest, such as body mass index and waist perimeter. This battery is an appropriate working tool for the operationalization of adapted exercise programs in the older adult, allowing the basal characterization of the individual and monitoring the effect of the exercise program on the improvement of individual capacities evaluated.

Benefits of exercise for health and aging

The benefits of regular and properly oriented exercise have been mentioned over the years. By way of example, Taylor and Johnson[29] refer to some of the major contributions, grouped into three areas, mainly physiological benefits, functional benefits, and other relevant benefits. Physiological benefits include increased maximum heart rate capacity for exercise, decreased heart rate at rest and during exercise, increased volume, increased blood circulation, increased muscle vascularization, increased oxygen extraction from muscle tissues, and increased capacity for maximum oxygen consumption. Regarding functional benefits, it includes increased efficiency in physical activity, decrease in muscle stress, increased maximum exercise capacity, and increased tolerance for submaximal activities at higher heart rates. Other benefits comprise decreased risk of early death, decreased risk of coronary heart disease, decreased risk of oncological disease (colon, breast), decreased risk of diabetes mellitus II, improved body composition, among others.

Regular physical activity is an important non-pharmacological aid in the treatment of depressive conditions in the older adult, as it promotes their commitment to a more active lifestyle associated with greater social interaction increasing self-esteem and self-confidence.

Discussion and conclusions

Despite the recommendations of the World Health Organization, and the worldwide awareness about the need to maintain active living habits in the older population, the real implementation of this endorsement is still far from desirable in several aspects, such as the coverage of the older population as a whole. Thus, there is an urgent need to build multidisciplinary teams including professionals specialized in exercise prescription for this particular population, working in an integrated way with the primary care and other relevant facilities of support to the elder population.

The rootedness of primary care in communities, and the close relationship that traditionally exists with the older population, is an important factor for the effectiveness of the implementation of physical exercise in the older adult, as well as other forms of structured intervention, understood in a holistic and multidisciplinary approach, as recommended in the AGA@4life model. In fact, it is within multidisciplinary primary care teams that more complete knowledge of the environment in which older people are inserted becomes more accessible, allowing for in-depth information on community resources (associations, groups of residents, among others), literacy, social, economic, and infrastructural aspects, in short, about all the ecological and contextual aspects that characterize the daily life of each older person. This knowledge would allow the planning, implementation, and management of physical exercise, individually, considering the specific needs of each person, and framed within the region in which the person lives.

The contribution of a course of action framed in the implementation of an intervention model such as AGA@4life, in proximity to the older adult, would also be expected at the level of global literacy regarding the importance of adopting healthy lifestyles, providing important tools for individual decision-making regarding commitment to one's own health, and to responsible participation and involvement in the health and integration of the older adult. Through this awareness, the necessary conditions would be created for each person to be able to integrate the need for physical exercise as a life activity, by the realization that this is effectively an important contribution to their health, and not just a task for which they are sometimes not motivated.

Key points

- Exercise is a key determinant of healthy and active aging.
- The practice of physical exercise in the older adult must be individually adapted to their functional capacity, individual needs, and available resources.
- Exercise in the older adult should be part of a multidisciplinary strategy for promoting healthy lifestyles.
- The AGA@4life Intervention Model is an integrated, multidisciplinary and personalized strategy for promoting active and healthy aging in which physical exercise plays a key role.

Notes

1. 1 MET – amount of energy used in resting state.
2. FITT – The acronym stands for Frequency, Intensity, Time, and Type.
3. 1RM – Corresponds to one repetition with the maximum load.

References

1 Fiatarone MA, O'Neill EF, Ryan ND, Clements KM, Solares GR, Nelson ME, Roberts SB, Kehayias JJ, Lipsitz LA, Evans WJ. Exercise training and nutritional supplementation for physical frailty in very elderly people. N Engl J Med. 1994;330(25):1769–75.

2 Instituto Nacional de Estatística. Estimativas de População Residente em Portugal 2018. 2018:1–13.

3 Serra e Silva P. Aprender a Não Ser Velho. Mar de Palavra, ed. 2012.

4 Ostir GV, Markides KS, Black SA, Goodwin JS. Emotional well-being predicts subsequent functional independence and survival. J Am Geriatr Soc. 2000;48(5):473–8.

5 Dias G, Mendes R, Serra e Silva P, Branquinho MA (2014). Envelhecimento Activo e Actividade Física. In: Gonçalo Dias, Rui Mendes, Polybio Serra e Silva, eds. Maria Aurora Banquinho. Coimbra. Escola Superior de Educação de Coimbra. 2014.

6 Ford AB, Folmar SJ, Salmon RB, Medalie JH, Roy AW, Galazka SS. Health and function in the old and very old. J Am Geriatr Soc. 1988;36(3):187–97.

7 Baumgartner RN. Body composition in healthy aging. Ann N Y Acad Sci. 2000;904:437–48.

8 Wang ZM, Pierson RN Jr, Heymsfield SB. The five-level model: a new approach to organizing body-composition research. Am J Clin Nutr. 1992;56(1):19–28.

9 Mazariegos M, Heymsfield SB, Wang ZM, Wang J, Yasumura S, Dilmanian FA, Pierson RN Jr. Aging affects body composition: young versus elderly women pair-matched by body mass index. Basic Life Sci. 1993;60:245–9.

10 Spirduso W, Macrae P, Francis K. Physical Dimensions of Aging. Champaign, IL: Human Kinetics Publishers. 2004.

11 Correia P, Silva A. Alterações da função neuromuscular no idoso. Atas do Simpósio 99, Envelhecer melhor com a actividade física. Cruz Quebrada: Edições da Faculdade de Motricidade Humana. 1999.

12 Singh MA. Exercise comes of age: rationale and recommendations for a geriatric exercise prescription. J Gerontol A Biol Sci Med Sci. 2002;57(5):M262–82.

13 Ascensão A, Magalhães J, Oliveira J, Duarte J, Soares J. Fisiologia da fadiga muscular. Delimitação conceptual, modelos de estudo e mecanismos de fadiga de origem central e periférica. Rev Port Ciências do Desporto. 2003;3(1):108–23.

14 Freitas EV, Miranda RD, Nery M. Parâmetros clínicos do envelhecimento e avaliação geriátrica global. In: Freitas E, Py L, Cançado F, Doll J, Gorzoni ML, organizadores. Tratado de geriatria e gerontologia. Rio de Janeiro: Guanabara-Koogan. 2002.

15 Terry RD, Katzman R. Life span and synapses: will there be a primary senile dementia? Neurobiol Aging. 2001;22:347–8.

16 Dickstein DL, Kabaso D, Rocher AB, Luebke JI, Wearne SL, Hof PR. Changes in the structural complexity of the aged brain. Aging Cell. 2007;6:275–84.

17 Martin J S, Jerger JF. Some effects of aging on central auditory processing. J Rehabil Res Dev. 2005;42(4):25–44.

18 Borges S de M, Cintra FA. Relação entre acuidade visual e atividades instrumentais de vida diária em idosos em seguimento ambulatorial. Rev Bras Oftalmol. 2010;69(3):146–51.

19 Antes D, Katzer J, Corazza S. Coordenação motora fina e propriocepção de idosas praticantes de hidroginástica. Revista Brasileira De Ciências Do Envelhecimento Humano. 2009;5(2):24–32.

20 World Health Organization. Global recommendations on physical activity for health. 2010.

21 Norman K. Exercise and Wellness for Older Adults. 2nd edition. Champaign, IL: Human Kinetics Publishers. 2010.

22 World Health Organization. Information sheet: global recommendations on physical activity for health 65 years and above. 2011.

23 Pescatello L, Arena R, Riebe D, Thompson P. ACSM's Guidelines for Exercise Testing and Prescription. 9th edition. Baltimore, ML: Lippincott Williams & Wilkins. 2013

24 Nelson ME, Rejeski WJ, Blair SN, Duncan PW, Judge JO, King AC, et al. Physical activity and public health in older adults: recommendation from the American College of Sports Medicine and the American Heart Association. Circulation. 2007;116(9):1094–105.

25 Borg G. Borg's Perceived Exertion and Pan Scales. Champaign, IL: Human Kinetics. 1998.

26 Zaleski AL, Taylor BA, Panza GA, et al. Coming of age: considerations in the prescription of exercise for older adults. Methodist Debakey Cardiovasc J. 2016;12(2):98–104.

27 Rikli RE, Jones CJ. Development and validation of a functional fitness test for community- residing older adults. J Aging Phys Act. 1999;7(2):129–61.

28 Rikli RE, Jones CJ. Development and validation of criterion-referenced clinically relevant fitness standards for maintaining physical independence in later years. Gerontologist. 2013;53(2):255–67.

29 Taylor A, Johnson M. Physiology of Exercise and Healthy Aging. Champaign, IL: Human Kinetics Publishers. 2008.

4 BrainAnswer platform

Biosignals acquisition for monitoring of physical and cardiac conditions of older people

João Valente, Veronika Kozlova, and Telmo Pereira

Introduction

The increase in the aging population and the consequent decrease in the active population lead to an imbalance of the demographic pyramid. According to *The 2012 Aging Report Economic and budgetary projections for the 27 EU Member States (2010–2060)* [1] it is estimated that the European population will reach 517 million by 2060 and the population over 65 will increase from 17% to 30%, the population between 15 and 64 years will fall from 67% to 56% and those under 15 years from 16% to 14% [1]. Recently published projections [2] indicate that in the EU in 2070, for every person over 65 there will be only two people of working age. These data lead us to look at the next decades with concern, as the various studies are unanimous, the demographic pyramid imbalance is a reality [2] and there are countries where this imbalance is coming about even faster [2, 3]. The model based on intergenerational solidarity where the active population guarantees the retirement of the older population is becoming less and less sustainable as the age pyramid changes. Extraordinary measures for the transfer of funds for social security or increasing retirement age are more and more common, but not sustainable in the long term [2]. The existence of increasingly aging societies generates a bigger need for health care that is not covered by the national health care systems and is often provided by informal caregivers. In Portugal, the Informal Caregiver Statute was recently approved, amending the Social Security Welfare Contributions Code [4]. However, resorting to informal caregivers creates other kinds of problems, for example, caregivers are essentially active women affecting the labor market and causing a partial or temporary loss of a worker. On the other hand, the ability to care often decreases over time due to the negative emotional impact that these tasks can have [2, 3].

DOI: 10.4324/9781003215271-4

With not enough people to treat people, it is urgent to look for new ways to act, make people more independent, ensure greater security at home, provide them with friendlier remote assistance resources, easier access to computer resources and provide adequate training for the older people and caregivers [5, 6]. We look at machines, robots [7, 8], artificial intelligence [9], the Internet of Things [10], the machine's ability to understand people's needs, ability to identify their emotions [11–13], and enhance the best response to their requests [14]. We are looking for robots with a "canine soul" always faithful to their owner, counteracting loneliness [15] with a nurse's hand, a doctor's mind [16], a listener to their memories, their voice as well as their children's and grandchildren's voice and the affection of the loved one. "Where is my humanoid robot Sofia?" [14]. How can we view demographic change? The hospital is changing and new tools, new technologies are emerging every day [17]. The digital age began long ago and so did its faults and benefits. We live connected to social networks, we seek the comfort of a LIKE [18, 19], we are swallowed up by this society of consumption, supply, and demand, which lives in immediacy, which feels pain when it logs off creating a phenomenon of silence, isolation, and loneliness [19, 20]. Let's also look at the benefits: being connected anytime and anywhere, accessing memories and past events, asking for help, working from home, meeting with people on the other side of the world, researching products, finding reviews, travel, offers, taking courses, and study. Learning a new profession through a course online, a new way to interact with the future, a new way to help ourselves in health and sickness. On the other hand, the older population needs differentiated care according to their physical condition and level of dependence: active, fragile or dependent, remote location, financial condition, difficulty in accessing health centers [21]. Older adult support concepts such as longer independent living, assisted living, long-term care [3], the silver economy [21], and many others are proliferating in an attempt to start the path back home from hospital or new ways to approach the older adult. The AGA@4Life project [22] seeks to study the older adult in all aspects, taking a broad geriatric approach where nothing is left out, where the person is the center of attention and where technology can be put at the service of the older adult. Thus comes the idea of using BrainAnswer [23], an online platform that facilitates the data collection process through the creation of dedicated protocols and simultaneous collection of physiological signals.

The broader objective of this work was to study the best way to create an adjustable dynamic for this population through a cyclic process of heart condition assessment and therapy adjustment. The first phase, which will be described in this chapter, was to create the material and human conditions for conducting an assessment of the heart condition of the older adult in their place of residence and ensuring good quality of the collected electrocardiogram (ECG) signal. Heart assessment was centered on heart rate variability (HRV) analysis metrics. In this sense the BrainAnswer platform was adapted taking into account the directives and guidelines for a good report based on HRV analysis [24, 25].

Testing the BrainAnswer platform

The BrainAnswer platform was used to construct the experimental paradigm and a low cost BiTalino equipment was used [26, 27] with a system of three electrodes: two differentials and a reference to obtain the ECG tracing. The BrainAnswer Client V0.16.0 application was used in the collection process, software that includes drivers' equipment, biosigns preview and sequential presentation of stimuli to participants. The sampling frequency used was 1000 Hz. Further feature extraction was performed using the BioSPPy toolbox, a set of open source and Python-based routines for ECG signal filtering, R-peak detection, Heart Rate (HR) plot, waveform template [28]. The BioSPPy toolbox applies a bandpass filter (3–45 Hz) and also implements Christov's algorithm for QRS detection [29].

Methods

The participants were at least 15 minutes in a relaxing room, then placed in the supine position and the electrode placement procedure was started. After verifying good signal quality, the protocol defined for this study was initiated, consisting of two forms, one with demographic data and questions related to the participants' clinical history and the other with the International Physical Activity Questionnaire (IPAQ) [30]. The technician was asking questions to the participants and introducing the information into the platform to keep the participants as relaxed as possible. After completing the questionnaire, data collection was started for 300 seconds, advised to obtain HRV data of 5 minutes.

Experimental design

The construction of the experimental design followed several steps from target audience definition to HRV report generation and described below.

Target population

Selecting the target population and verifying the conditions for admissibility to the study corresponds to an important step, either because the data collected do not serve the study or the participant's conditions make it impossible to apply all necessary procedures. An admissibility questionnaire is usually conducted and informed consent is given for self-authorization.

In the present study, samples of participants from the older adult and students had already been previously selected for the AGA@4LIFE project, and the ethical requirements for the research were verified at the outset. Acquisitions with students allowed the protocol procedures to be improved and validated, and collections with the older adult allowed them to assess their heart condition and out-of-lab acquisition method. In this sense, 20 participants from a day care center older than 65 were selected and 20 participants with a mean age of 21 years old.

Protocol

It corresponds to the definition of the elements that must be integrated in the construction of the paradigm and tasks to be performed by the participants. The BrainAnswer platform has an area reserved for the implementation of a new protocol. In the present case the constituent elements of the protocol were: The participant's demographic data form and some health indicators, Figure 4.1, the IPAQ form for physical activity level assessment, Figure 4.2, and the final ECG collection task during 5 minutes, Figure 4.3.

Sensor placement lace and specialized technicians for acquisition

Sensor placement procedures, verification of the required environmental conditions and the participant's physical and emotional conditions must be checked at the time of registration to ensure good signals are collected. Each piece of equipment used has very specific characteristics that should be well taken care of by experienced professionals or well-trained informal caregivers so as not to undermine the study. In the present study, all collections were performed by the same specialized technician. This ensured that the procedures were the same throughout the process. The place chosen for the collection of student data was a laboratory and the older adult nursing home.

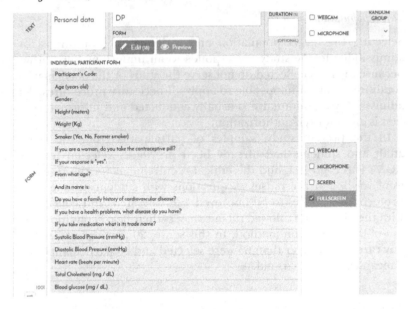

Figure 4.1 Demographics data platform implementation interface. Information to the participant about the demographic questionnaire and clinical situation of some parameters. The participant may continue or give up and the response time is not limited. Questionnaire response with no limited response time. The screen is fullscreen

Equipment

The BrainAnswer platform allows multiple data collection instruments to be used simultaneously or individually and multimodal studies can be performed, Figure 4.4. The technologies and equipment already tested and integrated are:

Forms
Bitalino based Biosense (ECG, GSR, RESP, and PULSE)
Screen record
Webcam
Emotiv (14 Channels)
Audio
Eye-tracker (GazePoint 120 Hz)
Mouse tracker
and in integration
Thermal camera (Optris PI 400/450)
EEG + Biosignals g.Nautilus

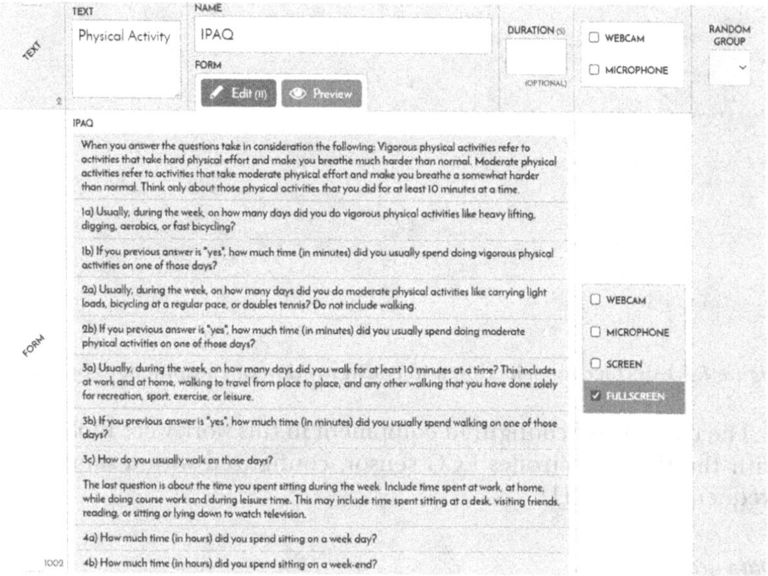

Figure 4.2 Platform interface for IPAQ placement. Information to the participant about physical activity questionnaire. Response time is not limited. The screen is fullscreen

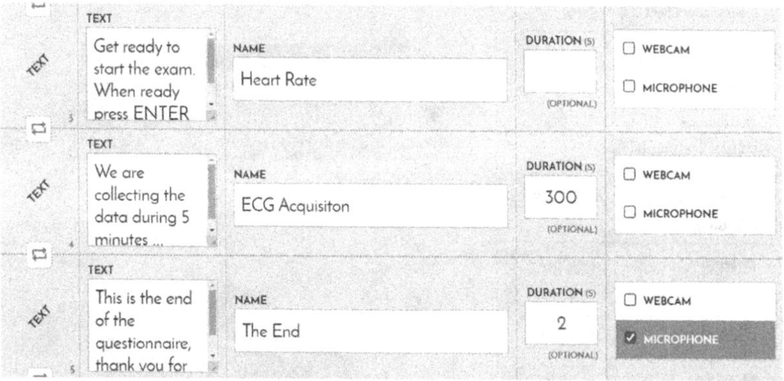

Figure 4.3 Platform interface for 300 seconds ECG acquisition time. Performing ECG Signal Collection: Information on the procedures to be taken into account during ECG registration and the conditions that must be observed during collection. The participant may continue or give up and the response time is not limited. ECG registration with fixed duration of 300 seconds. Registration ends with a thank you. The system returns a message if the data was submitted correctly

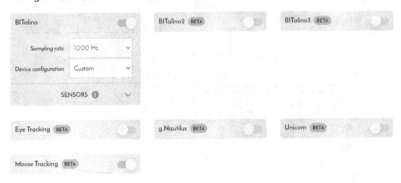

Figure 4.4 Interface for selection and configuration of equipment to be used

The chosen and configured equipment in this work were BioSense with the three electrodes ECG sensor, configured with a sampling frequency of 1000 Hz.

Data acquisition

Local data acquisition was performed with the BrainAnswer Client application. At first the protocol built for this study was discharged, the electrodes placed and the ECG signal visualized. This way it was possible to evaluate the signal quality, noise level or artifacts, Figure 4.5.

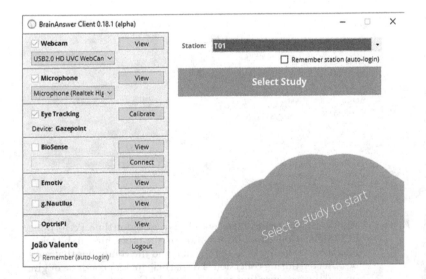

Figure 4.5 BrainAnswer Client

After this validation phase, data collection began. After the acquisition, the data were sent to the BrainAnswer platform where they were processed.

Data treatment

For the filtering and data processing procedures the BioSPPy tool was used [28]. The procedures used on the platform were:

1 Raw data preview synchronized with displayed stimuli. This makes it possible to visually validate the biosignals and in the particular case of this ECG study (Figure 4.6).
2 Visualization of the result of applying the filters to the ECG signal, to validate the signal quality and possible removal of artifacts (Figure 4.6b).
3 Visualization of the performance of the R wave detection algorithm to ensure that there are no flaws in determining the RR intervals (Figure 4.6b).
4 Visualization of the evolution of the heartbeat graph (Figure 4.6c).
5 Calculation of time, frequency, and nonlinear parameters for HRV assessment.
6 Presentation of HRV Individual Report.

A case study

Comparison of HRV parameters of old and young participant

In order to better demonstrate the tools available on the platform, the ECGs and some parameters extracted from the HRV report of two subjects will be compared (Figure 4.7). The older adult female participant (34), 70 years old, 1.45 m tall, 73 kg weight does not exercise and walks 4 times a week at a slow pace without causing breathing alteration and the young female participant (3) 18 years old, 1.7 m tall, 60 kg weight who does not exercise and walks every day approximately 15 minutes.

Making these tools available on the platform enables the necessary validation procedures recommended by the European guidelines [24, 25], possibility of visualizing raw data, visualization of the filter application results and confirmation of the good performance of the R wave detection algorithm.

The main variables of the cardiovascular system are influenced by the autonomic nervous system (ANS), which is considered an

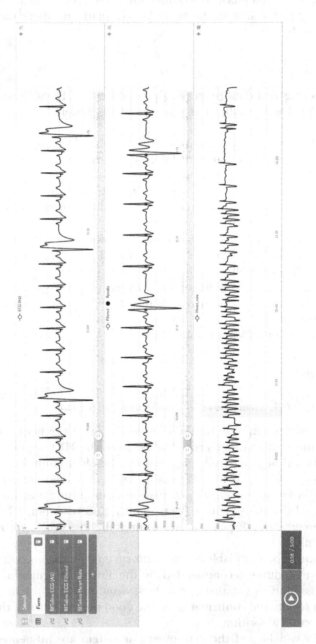

Figure 4.6 Raw data Treatment: (a) Acquired ECG signal, top graph. (b) Filtered signal and location/marking with R wave points, middle graph. (c) Heart rate estimation, graph below

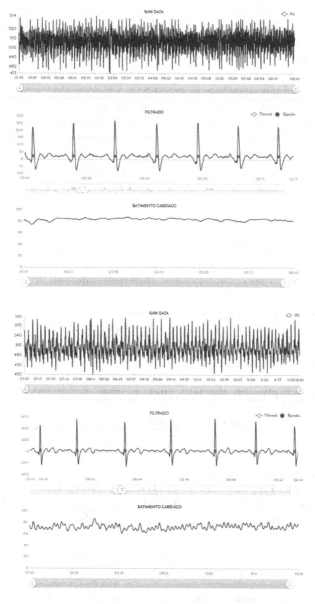

Figure 4.7 Display of participant (34) left side and participant (3) right side signals. The graphs above correspond to the raw signal, the middle signals correspond to the filtered ECG signal and the R wave markers (yellow dots) are calculated by the algorithm. The graph below corresponds to the variation of each participant's heartbeat

important modulator of cardiovascular function and is directly correlated with HRV. Sympathovagal balance is influenced by various factors such as weight, age, gender [31], physical activity, family history, illness, medication [32] and others. It is often not easy to identify whether this is more related to increased sympathetic activity or to decreased parasympathetic activity.

The sympathetic nervous system constantly acts to modulate the functioning of various organ systems, such as the heart, blood vessels, the gastrointestinal tract, the bronchi and the sweat glands. On the other hand, the parasympathetic nervous system acts through the vagus nerve.

R-R interval variations are used for the analysis of time and frequency domain indices and nonlinear methods.

Time domain analysis of HRV parameters

For time domain analysis, the indices obtained use time as a variable (ms – milliseconds) and certain statistical or geometric procedures are applied to successive normal interbeat intervals that analyze HRV. Thus, the translating indices of autonomic fluctuations in the duration of the cardiac cycles are calculated.

The RMSSD and pNN50 indices represent parasympathetic activity and can be analyzed in short-term collections for example 5 minutes. The SDNN index is more associated with the sympathetic and parasympathetic systems.

Figure 4.8 presents the HRV time analysis parameters extracted from the RR interval series. On the left column are the data of an older adult participant and on the right column a younger participant.

Some parameters of HRV on time domain are summarized in Table 4.1.

From the analysis of the results obtained from the parameters of time domain, it is possible to see that in the older adult participant all indicators reflect a decrease in HRV, the higher HR may be related to overweight. All other indicators are smaller for the young participant (Figure 4.8, Table 4.1).

Frequency domain analysis of HRV parameters

The frequency domain analysis is extracted from the Fourier transform of the time-resampled HR signal. The main components of this analysis are: the high frequency (HF) component, ranging from 0.15 to 0.4 Hz, indicating vagus nerve activity over the heart; low

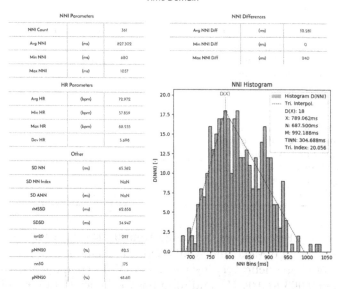

Figure 4.8 HRV time parameters and histogram nni (a) participant (34), older adult, left side and (b) participant (3) young, right side

Table 4.1 Comparison of HRV time parameters for older adult and young participant

HRV parameters	Old participant (34)	Young participant (3)
Average HR (bpm) – Standard deviation HR	83.53–2.17	72.97–5.70
SDNN – Standard deviation of all NN intervals (ms)	19.35	65.36
RMSSD – The square root of the mean of the sum of the squares of differences between adjacent NN intervals (ms)	11.57	62.86
SDSD – Standard deviation of differences between adjacent NN intervals (ms)	7.01	34.95
NN20 – Number of pairs of adjacent NN intervals differing by less than 20 ms in the entire recording. pNN20 % de NN	29 (7%)	297 (82.5%)
NN50 – Number of pairs of adjacent NN intervals differing by more than 50 ms in the entire recording. pNN50 % de NN	0 (0%)	175 (48.6%)
HRV triangular index – Total number of all NN intervals divided by the height of the histogram of all NN intervals measured on a discrete scale with bins of 7·8125 ms (1/128 s).	4.837	20.056
TINN-Baseline width of the minimum square difference triangular interpolation of the highest peak of the histogram of all NN intervals (ms)	62.500	304.688

frequency (LF) component, ranging from 0.04 to 0.15 Hz, due to the joint action of vagal and sympathetic modulation, with predominance of sympathetic; very low frequency (VLF) components, ranging from 0.003 to 0.04 Hz, and ultra low frequency (ULF), ranging <0.003 Hz, whose physiological explanation is not well understood. The LF/HF ratio characterizes the sympathovagal balance over the heart [33].

In the spectral analysis of HRV parameters (Figure 4.9, Table 4.2) that were performed in absolute values and normalized units, the older participant had a higher LF (nu) 84.365 versus 29.014 component, indicating that there is a greater predominance of the sympathetic component, lower HF (nu) (15,635 versus 70,986), indicating a very low level of parasympathetic activation and high LF/HF (5,396 versus 0.409), indicating worse sympathovagal imbalance compared to the young participant.

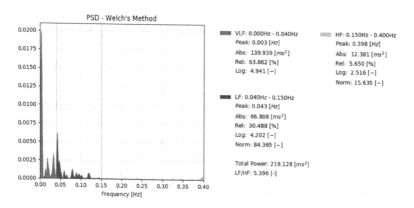

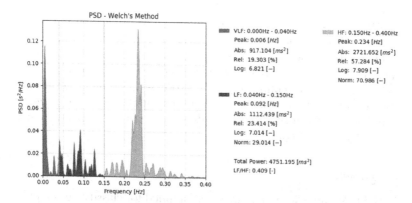

Figure 4.9 Spectral result of HRV parameters (a) of the older participant and (b) of the younger participant

Table 4.2 Comparison of HRV frequency parameters for older adult and young participant

HRV frequency parameters	Old participant (34)	Young participant (3)
LF(nu)	84.365	29.014
HF (nu)	15.635	70.986
LF/HF	5.396	0.409

Nonlinear HRV parameters

Nonlinear analytical methods were applied to identify HRV-associated parameters indicative of changes in autonomic modulation of cardiac function.

A Poincaré plot is a scatter plot of RR_n vs. RR_{n+1} where RR_n is the time between two successive R peaks and RR_{n+1} is the time between the next two successive R peaks. When the plot is adjusted by the ellipse fit method, the analysis provides three indices: the standard deviation of the instantaneous beat-to-beat interval variability (SD1), the long-term variability of the continuous RR intervals (SD2), and the ratio SD1/SD2 (SD12). In Poincaré's plot, SD1 is the width and SD2 is the length of the ellipse [34].

SD1 has been shown to correlate with short-term HRV and is mainly influenced by parasympathetic modulation, whereas SD2 is a measure of long-term variability and reflects sympathetic activation [34].

From the visual analysis of the Poincaré graph (Figure 4.10) the older adult participant showed less dispersion of RR intervals, both between two successive R peaks, and long term indicating a decrease in the older adult participant's HRV.

SD1 was lower in the older adult (Figure 4.10) indicating that parasympathetic regulation is weakened by age and probably by overweight.

The alpha 1 and alpha 2 values of the *older adult* are higher than those of the young and may also be related to age (Figure 4.10).

Note that we are comparing only two cases, one older adult and one young, so these results cannot be extrapolated to the general population without conducting studies with many more participants and free of pathologies.

IPAQ results

To the IPAQ questionnaire rules were applied for classifying the participants' physical activity level (high, low, and moderate) according to their answers.

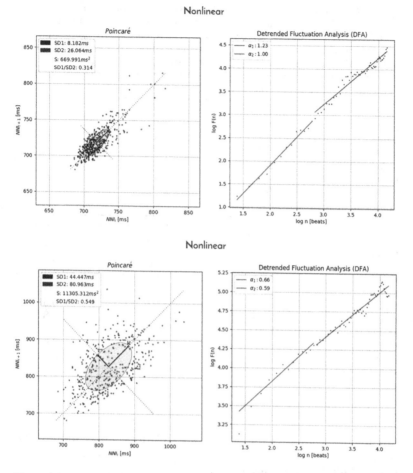

Figure 4.10 Parameters obtained from nonlinear analysis. SD1, SD2, and SD1/SD2 ratios obtained from Poincaré plot

Looking at the first column of Table 4.3, we find that in this particular case there are no differences between the two groups, the pattern of physical exercise is too similar between the sample of students and the sample of older adult in the day care center.

From the observation of the second column, the pattern in Table 4.3 is equally similar, with a small difference in the performance of more intense physical exercises, that is, the young group performs more intense exercise per week.

Table 4.3 Summary display of the IPAQ classification for physical activity. Left table represents the absolute and relative frequencies according to group (old versus young) and level of physical activity (high, moderate, and low). Right table depicts the weekly averages for hours of exercise (Avg HE), number of days of exercise (Avg DE) and sitting hours (Avg HS)

Class	Count	%
OLD	20	
High	1	5%
Low	16	80%
Moderate	3	15%
Young	20	
High	1	5%
Low	14	70%
Moderate	5	25%

Class	Avg HE	Avg DE	Avg HS
High	**8.8**	**6.5**	**5.1**
Old	5.8	4.0	4.7
Young	11.7	9.0	5.4
Low	**2.4**	**2.9**	**6.5**
Old	2.2	2.4	6.3
Young	2.7	3.6	6.8
Moderate	**8.2**	**6.3**	**5.4**
Old	9.5	6.0	6.0
Young	7.5	6.4	5.1

Conclusion

Preliminary analysis of the BrainAnswer platform application to the study of the older adult in their usual ecosystem revealed that it presents the minimum requirements to be used as an ECG data collection instrument for the assessment of heart condition and the monitoring of the application of personalized programs of physical exercise.

The possibility of implementing experimental protocols that include forms, different equipment, task timing, scheduling of interventions, among other features, allows one to carry out screening programs and remote evaluation of cardiac condition parameters. The provision of heart rate variation parameters also offers a clinical management tool that enables the definition of safe heart rate thresholds during training, as well as the monitoring of fitness from a cardiovascular perspective, in view of the availability of parameters, which express the influence of the Sympathetic Nervous System, the Parasympathetic Nervous System and the balance between them.

Since this is not a Life Support System, the remote signal quality validation tools obtained from raw signals, filtered signals and RR interval identification algorithms allow platform users to validate remotely acquired signals. The implementation of HRV parameter extraction algorithms and their graphical representation further support new studies in this area of knowledge. In this way, we think we are contributing to the implementation of mechanisms that can accompany older populations who are far from health centers by providing them with non-urgent clinical support, avoiding unnecessary travel, reducing discomfort, transportation expenses and allowing a history of patient follow-up. In future work we intend to implement therapeutic prescription protocols applied to each particular individual.

Key points

- Remote monitoring is a promising approach to ensure point-of-care vigilance in an aging society.
- The BrainAnswer platform is a feasible tool to monitor the heart condition of the older adult in its usual ecosystem.
- The BrainAnswer platform provides tools to monitor and assist in the implementation of tailored physical exercise programs.

References

1 E. C. D.-G. Economic & F. A. E. P. C. A. W. Group, "The 2012 Ageing Report: Economic and budgetary projections for the 27 EU Member States (2010–2060)," 2012.

2 E. C. D.-G. Economic & F. A. E. P. C. A. W. Group, "The 2018 Ageing Report: Economic and budgetary projections for the 28 EU Member States (2016–2070). Institutional Paper 079," 2018.

3 OECD. "Health at a Glance 2017 OECD INDICATORS". Tech. rep., OECD Publishing, 2017.

4 Lei n.º 100/2019 Diário da República n.º 171/2019, Série I de 2019-09-06, 2019.

5 L. Probst, L. Frideres, B. Pedersen, J.B. Marchive, & P. Luxembourg., P. (2015). "Independent living Case study 47," 2015.

6 L. Probst, L. Frideres, B. Pedersen, J. Bolanowska & C. Marchive, "Active aging Case study 48," 2015.

7 B.-J. Krings & N. Weinberger, "Assistant without Master? Some Conceptual Implications of Assistive Robotics in Health Care," *Technologies*, vol. 6, 1, p. 13, 2018.

8 K. Cresswell, S. Cunningham-Burley & A. Sheikh, "Health Care Robotics: Qualitative Exploration of Key Challenges and Future Directions," *Journal of Medical Internet Research*, vol. 20, 7, p. e10410, 2018.

9 L. G. Pee, S. L. Pan & L. Cui, "Artificial Intelligence in Healthcare Robots: A Social Informatics Study of Knowledge Embodiment," *Journal of the Association for Information Science and Technology*, vol. 70, 12, pp. 351–369, 2018.

10 S. M. R. Islam, D. Kwak, M. H. Kabir, M. Hossain & K.-S. Kwak, "The Internet of Things for Health Care: A Comprehensive Survey," *IEEE Access*, vol. 3, pp. 678–708, 2015.

11 J. James, C. I. Watson & B. MacDonald, "Artificial Empathy in Social Robots: An Analysis of Emotions in Speech," In: *2018 27th IEEE International Symposium on Robot and Human Interactive Communication (RO-MAN)*, 2018.

12 P. Dachkinov, T. Tanev, A. Lekova, D. Batbaatar & H. Wagatsuma, "Design and Motion Capabilities of an Emotion-Expressive Robot EmoSan," In: *2018 Joint 10th International Conference on Soft Computing and Intelligent Systems (SCIS) and 19th International Symposium on Advanced Intelligent Systems (ISIS)*, 2018.

13 M. Anjum, "Emotion Recognition from Speech for an Interactive Robot Agent," In: *2019 IEEE/SICE International Symposium on System Integration (SII)*, 2019.

14 A. Joseph, B. Christian, A. A. Abiodun & F. Oyawale, "A Review on Humanoid Robotics in Healthcare," *MATEC Web of Conferences*, vol. 153, p. 02004, 2018.

15 C. Huisman & H. Kort, "Two-Year Use of Care Robot Zora in Dutch Nursing Homes: An Evaluation Study," *Healthcare*, vol. 7, 2, p. 31, 2019.

16 E. D. Oña, J. M. Garcia-Haro, A. Jardón & C. Balaguer, "Robotics in Health Care: Perspectives of Robot-Aided Interventions in Clinical Practice for Rehabilitation of Upper Limbs," *Applied Sciences*, vol. 9, 6, p. 2586, 2019.

17 M. Vatandsoost & S. Litkouhi, "The Future of Healthcare Facilities: How Technology and Medical Advances May Shape Hospitals of the Future," *Hospital Practices and Research*, vol. 4, 2, pp. 1–11, 2019.

18 H. Odacı & Ç. B. Çelik, "Does Internet Dependence Affect Young Peoples Psycho-Social Status? Intrafamilial and Social Relations, Impulse Control, Coping Ability and Body Image," *Computers in Human Behavior*, vol. 57, 4, pp. 343–347, 2016.

19 R. Yavich, N. Davidovitch & Z. Frenkel, "Social Media and Loneliness – Forever Connected?," *Higher Education Studies*, vol. 9, 2, p. 10, 2019.

20 N. Bayindir & D. Kavanagh, "Social: The latest trends in social media. GlobalWebIndex's flagship report 2018," 2018.

21 E. Commission, "Growing the European Silver Economy," 2015.

22 T. Pereira, Abordagem Geriátrica Ampla Na Promoção de Um Envelhecimento Ativo e Saudável., I. P. Coimbra IPC | Inovar Para Crescer, Ed., SerSilito – Empresa Gráfica, Lda. – Maia, 2019.

23 BrainAnswer, "Homepage BrainAnswer, www.brainanswer.pt," last accessed 2019/10/01.

24 Marek Malik, "Guidelines Heart Rate Variability Standards of Measurement, Physiological Interpretation, and Clinical Use Task Force of The European Society of Cardiology and The North American Society of Pacing and Electrophysiology," *European Heart Journal*, vol. 17, pp. 354–381, 1996.

25 D. S. Quintana, G. A. Alvares & J. A. J. Heathers, "Guidelines for Reporting Articles on Psychiatry and Heart rate variability (GRAPH): Recommendations to Advance Research Communication," *Translational Psychiatry*, vol. 6, 5, pp. e803–e803, 2016.

26 "BITtalino: A Biosignal Acquisition System based on the Arduino," In: *Proceedings of the International Conference on Biomedical Electronics and Devices*, 2013.

27 "BITalino – A Multimodal Platform for Physiological Computing," In: *Proceedings of the 10th International Conference on Informatics in Control, Automation and Robotics*, 2013.

28 I. Telecomunicacoes, "BioSPPy Documentation, Release 0.6.1," 2018.

29 I. I. Christov, "Real Time Electrocardiogram QRS Detection Using Combined Adaptive Threshold," *BioMedical Engineering Online*, vol. 3, p. 28, 2004.

30 I. P. A. Q. R. Committee., "Guidelines for Data Processing and Analysis of the International Physical Activity Questionnaire (IPAQ) – Short and Long Forms," 2005.

31 G. D. Spina, B. B. Gonze, A. C. B. Barbosa, E. F. Sperandio & V. Z. Dourado, "Presence of Age- and Sex-Related Differences in Heart Rate Variability Despite the Maintenance of a Suitable Level of Accelerometer-Based Physical Activity," *Brazilian Journal of Medical and Biological Research*, vol. 52, p. e8088, 2019.

32 J. A. Vitale, M. Bonato, A. L. L. Torre & G. Banfi, "Heart Rate Variability in Sport Performance: Do Time of Day and Chronotype Play A Role?," *Journal of Clinical Medicine*, vol. 8, 5, p. 723, 2019.

33 J. C. F. Sá, E. C. Costa, E. Silva & G. D. Azevedo, "Variabilidade da frequência cardíaca como método de avaliação do sistema nervoso autônomo na síndrome dos ovários policísticos," *Revista Brasileira de Ginecologia e Obstetrícia*, vol. 35, 9, pp. 421–426, 2013.

34 B. Roy & S. Ghatak, "Nonlinear Methods to Assess Changes in Heart Rate Variability in Type 2 Diabetic Patients," *Arquivos Brasileiros de Cardiologia*, vol. 101,4, pp.317–327, 2013.

5 Nutrition in aging

Maria Helena Loureiro

Introduction

The increasing number of older adults is a reality worldwide, and today there are 400 million old adults across the globe, a number that is predicted to rise to over 1000 million in 2020. Throughout history, one of the greatest concerns of Man has been the search for an extended life-span. Undoubtedly, this has happened due to scientific and technological progress which, although not equally distributed, has made mortality decrease, increasing quality of life.[1,2] Aging, health and nutrition are closely related. Nutritional status is assessed according to past and present food habits, with a special attention to nutrition in adult age.

Aging

Aging is universal. Old age can be defined as a step in life that follows maturity, and presents specific effects on the human body as the years go by. Chronologically, it is hard to define, as it depends on the socioeconomic growth of each society, and their members will present signs of aging, with limitations and loss of resilience, in different chronological ages.

The aging tendency of the Portuguese population is not far from the European picture and other countries, with similar socioeconomic characteristics, typified by a decrease in fertility and increased life-span. This is not unique to Portugal, but will surely continue, and so global action to promote healthy aging is necessary. According to the National Statistical Institute 2011 census, the aging index has increased from 102 in 2001, to 128 in 2011.[2] As an established phenomenon, aging comes from a determined growing and maturation process, that is unique to each individual. These differences are,

DOI: 10.4324/9781003215271-5

in part, genetically predetermined, but also influenced by lifestyle, environment and nutritional status. Nutrition plays a role not only in ensuring life but in maintaining optimal health status. According to the same author,[3] adequate nutrition for older adults is not very different from adults' in general, however, certain characteristics of aging, particular to older adults, determine different approaches to geriatric nutrition.[3]

There are a series of causes that promote malnutrition in the older adult:

- Low socioeconomic status;
- Disease;
- Decreased functional capacity;
- Low nutrition literacy;
- Inadequate food intake;
- Inability to cook and eat;
- Food habits and skipping meals;
- Social isolation;
- Loneliness;
- Physiological deficiencies;
- Alcohol;
- Depression and dependency;
- Physical restrictions;
- Inadequate medical prescriptions;
- Food beliefs;
- Institutionalization and others.

All of these facts contribute to malnutrition being present in a high percentage of older adults. On the other hand, malnutrition negatively influences the aging process, which is cause-independent. Older adults are frequently malnourished or obese, or with multiple nutrient deficiencies, which significantly contributes to complications, such as infections, pressure wounds, worsening of chronical disease and cognitive decline, which is explained by their vulnerability. Prevention and treatment of malnutrition are important goals in clinical nutrition. An early and precise diagnosis is essential for nutrition therapy to be initiated as soon as possible.

The increasing number of older adults is a universal reality. The aging process is highly complex and all its physiological aspects should be thoroughly analyzed. This might be understood as a progressive and dynamic process, in which there are morphological, functional and biochemical changes, which progressively alter the organism making it more susceptible to extrinsic and intrinsic aggressions, and leading to changes in the extracellular matrix, cell, tissues and organs.[4]

Aging happens across the life cycle and is due to genetic, hereditary, environmental, life and food habits. Aging does not happen equally to everyone, as we can see in completely dependent or independent older adults, which might happen due to sarcopenia. Due to the aging process, other limitations might occur, with consequences in food intake and nutritional status. In older adults, inadequate food intake added to a sedentary lifestyle results in degenerative and metabolic diseases.

Nutritional risk screening

Nutritional screening is essential and should be performed as early as possible, specifically in institutionalized and hospitalized older adults, which now is a quality standard in hospital care. Early recognition leads to an adequate and timely intervention. The method for nutritional risk screening should be quick, easy to apply and understand, non-invasive, and inexpensive. On the other hand, it should be specific, sensitive and with positive predictive value, diminishing the number of false positive and false negative results.[5] Its main purpose is to screen patients for nutritional risk and further apply specific assessment techniques to determine risk and establish an action plan. After screening, nutritional assessment follows, which determines the nutritional status through clinical, nutrition and social history, anthropometric data, biochemical data and drug-nutrient interactions, allowing one to classify the degree of malnutrition and define nutritional support and a monitoring plan.[5]

There are various tools to determine nutritional risk. The *Mini Nutritional Assessment* – MNA is one of the most used in this population[6] and validated in many countries, and in Portugal.[7] The MNA entails objective and subjective methods, both measurements and simple questions, and can be applied in less than 10 minutes:

- Anthropometric assessment (weight, height, arm, and calf circumference);
- Global assessment (lifestyle, medication, and mobility);
- Nutritional assessment (number of meals, food intake, and feeding independence);
- Subjective assessment (Self-perception of health and nutritional status).

Each item is scored and its total allows classification of nutritional status in older adults as adequate, or at risk of malnutrition and malnourished.[8]

Recommendations to older adults will be given according to the results: monitoring, nutritional assessment and/or nutritional intervention. This too has been developed specifically for older adults and appears to have higher sensitivity and specificity. MNA can identify risk of malnutrition in older adults before clinical manifestations emerge. It is a useful tool for Nutritionists, Physicians and Nurses, to quickly assess older adults as part of a global geriatric assessment and to recognize risk early on.

In the early nineties, Vellas et al.[9] developed MNA, which is easy to apply, quick and inexpensive, and allows one to assess nutritional status of older adults upon hospital admission, and to monitor changes that happen during a hospital stay. This makes nutritional therapy easy to implement early on, to prevent nutritional status decline. It is also used in institutionalized and for community-dwelling older adults.[10] The purpose of this is to determine the risk of malnutrition and allow a timely nutritional intervention.[9] The MNA is a non-invasive, practical tool, which allows a brief assessment of potential risk of malnutrition in older adults.

Nutritional status assessment

Malnutrition may be the result of an excess, deficit or imbalance of nutrients and energy that can exacerbate the nutritional status of older people.

Inadequate nutritional status contributes significantly to increased mortality, worsens the prognosis of older people with acute illness, and increases the use of hospitalization and institutionalization. With age there is a decrease in the mechanisms of ingestion, absorption, digestion, transport and excretion, which translates into specific needs in this stage of the life cycle.[11,12]

The incidence of malnutrition reaches significant levels in the older adult and should therefore be systematically identified and corrected. It is unanimous that nutritional assessment is a key parameter in comprehensive geriatric assessment.

Malnutrition in the older adult increases physical disability decreasing quality of life and increases morbidity and consequent mortality. It is often underdiagnosed, thus compromising an early recognition that would lead to timely readjustments. The most common causes are poor diet and increased needs. It is very important to identify the severity of malnutrition, since this is a complex problem, has a high prevalence, and needs immediate intervention. Malnutrition is the most worrisome and most common deviation in the geriatric population today; however, obesity should also be taken into account, as it is associated with various problems that influence the health of the older adult.

Assessing the nutritional status of the older population requires clinical assessment to detect physical signs of nutritional imbalances, studies to assess nutrient intake with recognized standards, laboratory research to obtain data on the amount of nutrients in the body or to assess certain biochemical functions that depend on adequate intake, and anthropometric assessment. The assessment of nutritional status cannot be performed with a single instrument because none have sufficient sensitivity or specificity to allow the diagnosis of the type and severity of malnutrition. Thus, for a correct evaluation it is necessary to associate several parameters, such as anthropometric, food intake, and biochemical data.[5]

Given that the use of a simple measure is insufficient to diagnose a level of malnutrition in a population as well as in the individual, it is essential to combine various methods. Assessing the nutritional status of individuals is a difficult and complex task given the numerous changes associated with aging that interfere with the commonly used nutritional assessment parameters. This can be done at four levels: clinical and functional assessment, food intake assessment, anthropometric and body composition assessment and biochemical assessment.

There are many proposed methods:

- Clinical history and physical examination;
- Food history;
- Anthropometry;
- Laboratory evaluation;
- Bioimpedance;
- Densitometry;
- MRI;
- CT scan;
- Others....

There is no perfect method; all have limitations often inherent to the method, other than inherent to the older adult. However, if we could have an ideal method, it would have to be: specific for nutritional status; sensitive to variations in nutritional status; reproducible; easily applicable; easily measurable; economic; accessible; fast.

The concept that the nutritional status of older individuals is the key factor of healthy aging has been proven by numerous studies.[13]

Sarcopenia is a progressive and generalized skeletal muscle disorder that is associated with an increased likelihood of falls, fractures, physical disability and mortality. In the 2018 definition, the European Group for the Study of Sarcopenia considers low muscle strength as the primary parameter of sarcopenia.[14] The diagnosis is confirmed by the presence of low muscle quantity or low muscle quality. When low muscle strength, low muscle quantity/quality, and poor physical performance are present, sarcopenia is considered severe.[14] Early onset sarcopenia leads to progressive disability and loss of independence. Skeletal muscle mass decreases by almost 50% between the ages of 20 and 90, by a percentage of 15% per decade starting at age 50 and about 30% per decade at 70 years of age. Aging itself triggers several mechanisms such as: increased oxidative stress due to free radical accumulation, physical inactivity and inadequate nutritional intake; increased apoptosis and mitochondrial dysfunction in myocytes; neurodegenerative processes; reduced anabolic hormone levels (testosterone, estrogens, GH, IGF-1); increased production of proinflammatory cytokines (TNF, IL-6). All of which contribute to the development of sarcopenia.[15,16] Of all these factors, sedentary lifestyle, physical inactivity and inadequate nutritional intake, despite their being related to the main cellular mechanisms underlying sarcopenia, they are modifiable factors and are especially prominent as an intervention strategy to reduce its progression.

Nutritional needs and maintaining proper nutrition

The eating plan for the older adult has to be customized and adapted to ensure adequate energy intake to meet macro and micronutrient needs and maintain adequate body weight.[17,18] With increasing age, nutritional needs are increased due to impaired absorption and effective utilization of certain nutrients.[17] Major aspects to consider are the total number of calories ingested, the distribution of calories throughout the day, the food sources that contribute to this caloric intake, the social and cultural aspects and the respect for individual tastes. Individualized nutritional intervention should ensure quality and protein density through healthy eating, taking into account all physiological and non-physiological factors that interfere with the older adult's food intake. It should also encompass the recommendation of meals at regular intervals respecting eating habits and taking into account dietary restrictions, according to the pathologies and organic dysfunctions.

Energy requirements may eventually decrease due to a possible decrease in physical activity and the consequent reduction in muscle mass. But most micronutrient requirements (vitamins and minerals) may even increase. In order to optimize the nutritional status we must take into account the indications of a healthy, varied and adapted diet, taking into account comorbidities and consequent medication, and the limitations that are inherent to aging, such as chewing difficulties, poorly adapted prostheses and the lack of teeth. Adaptations and modifications of textures in the eating plan are recommended in order to preserve the pleasantness. Also, the importance of chewing as a stimulation for the brain hippocampus should be acknowledge, considering its importance for the maintenance of memory and learning functions.[17] Culinary confections should promote digestibility and appetite (appearance, color, texture, aroma). Moisturizing is also extremely important, therefore promoting a proper water intake (about 8 glasses/day) is mandatory. Water can be flavored with fruits (lemon, orange) or be taken as cold herbal infusion tea (linden, lemon balm, mint), according to the individual specificities. The importance of hydration increases with age due to decreased renal function and decreased perception of thirst.[19]

Aging is also characterized by changes in the senses of taste and thirst, as well as changes in the jaws and dentition. All of these phenomena are unavoidable, but if detected and treated in a timely manner they will not have a significant impact on either the state of nutrition or the deterioration of the whole organism.

Conclusions

The World Health Organization (WHO) describes the quality of life associated with aging as a "broad and subjective concept that includes physical health, psychological status, degree of independence, social relationships, personal beliefs, and its relationship to important aspects of the environment."[20]

With the increase in life expectancy, it is important to join efforts so that this extended lifespan corresponds to a healthy and active status, so that the older adult can live each day independently in their daily tasks. Age-dependent changes, which have an expression in weight loss, anorexia and sarcopenia, can lead to frailty, which is associated with increased morbidity, decreased quality of life and institutionalization. The health systems, the professionals, the caregivers, the family and the community must join efforts to promote the adoption of healthy behaviors in order to allow the integration of the older adult in the society, as well as to support the individual's aging and its weaknesses and changes.[17] All of this may not lead to an exponential increase in the average life expectancy of the older adult, but it will surely extend their life years with better health and quality of life. It is urgent to know how to take care and intervene with the older population to improve health and their quality of life.

Key points

- Nutritional screening to identify older adult at nutritional risk is of paramount importance.
- Nutritional Assessment can classify the degree of malnutrition and monitor nutritional interventions.
- Nutritional intervention must be tailored to prevent malnutrition and improve quality of life.

References

1 Alencar, Raimunda Silva. O Envelhecimento em Questão. Informativo da Associação dos Aposentados da CEPLAC. Ano V. 2001.

2 INE censos 2011 Resultados definitivos – Portugal 2012. Instituto Nacional de Estatística, I.P. 2012.

3 Malcata F. O Idoso, a Nutrição e a Sociedade: considerações sobre quantidade e qualidade de vida. Geriatria. Geriatria. 2003;151(15):23–37.

4 Partridge L, Deelen J, Slagboom PE. Facing up to the global challenges of ageing. Nature. 2018;561(7721):45–56.

5 Ferry M, Alix E, Brocker P, Constans T, Lesourd B, Mischlich D, Pfitzenmeyer P, Vellas B. Nutrição da Pessoa Idosa Aspetos fundamentais, clínicos e psicossociais. 2nd ed. Lusociência, Loures. 2004.

6 Guigoz Y, Vellas B, Garry PJ. The mini nutritional assessment: a practical assessment tool for grading the nutritional state of elderly patients. In: Vellas B, Ed. The Mini Nutritional Assessment (MNA). Serdi Publisher, Paris. 1994.

7 Loureiro H. Validação do mini-nutritional assesment em idosos, tese de mestrado. Faculdade de Medicina da Universidade de Coimbra, Coimbra. 2014.

8 Guigoz Y, Vellas B. A Mini Avaliação Nutricional na Classificação do Estado Nutricional do Paciente Idoso: Apresentação, História e Validação do MNA. Nestlé. 2001.

9 Vellas B, Villars H, Abellan G, Soto ME, Rolland Y, Guigoz Y, Morley JE, Chumlea W, Salva A, Rubenstein LZ, Garry P. Overview of the MNA—its history and challenges. J Nutr Health Aging. 2006;10:456–63.

10 Vellas B, Guigoz Y, Garry PJ, Nourhashemi F, Bennahum D, Lauque S, Albarede JL. The Mini Nutritional Assessment (MNA) and its use in grading the nutritional state of elderly patients. Nutrition. 1999;15(2):116–22.

11 Sociedade Portuguesa de Geriatria e Gerontologia, Associação portuguesa de Nutricionistas. Alimentação do ciclo de vida, alimentação da pessoa idosa. Colecção E-books APN: n°31. 2013.

12 Rodrigues SS, Franchini B, Graça P, de Almeida MD. A new food guide for the Portuguese population: development and technical considerations. J Nutr Educ Behav. 2006;38(3):189–95.

13 Vellas BJ, Garry PJ. Aging and nutrition. In: Richard Ziegler, L.J. Filer Eds. Present Knowledge in Nutrition. 7th Ed. ILSI – Nutrition Foundation, Washington. 1996.

14 Cruz-Jentoft AJ, Bahat G, Bauer J, Boirie Y, Bruyère O, Cederholm T, Cooper C, Landi F, Rolland Y, Sayer AA, Schneider SM, Sieber CC, Topinkova E, Vandewoude M, Visser M, Zamboni M; Writing Group for the European Working Group on Sarcopenia in Older People 2 (EWGSOP2), and the Extended Group for EWGSOP2. Sarcopenia: revised European consensus on definition and diagnosis. Published online. 2018 Sep 24. doi: 10.1093/ageing/afy169

15 Roubenoff R, Hughes VA. Sarcopenia: current concepts. J Gerontol A Biol Sci Med Sci. 2000;55:M716–24.

16 Zhong S, Chen CN, Thompson LV. Sarcopenia of ageing: functional, structural and biochemical alterations. Rev Bras Fisioter. 2007;11(2):91–7.

17 Afonso C, Morais C, de Almeida MDV. Alimentação e Nutrição. In: Constança Paul, Óscar Ribeiro Eds. Manual de Gerontologia – Aspectos biocomportamentais, psicológicos e sociais do envelhecimento. Lidel, Lisbon. 2012.

18 Mahan L, Escott-Stump S. Krause – Alimentos, Nutrição e Dietoterapia. 12a edição. Saunders Elsevier, Philadelphia, PA. 2010.

19 Direção Geral da Saúde. Programa Nacional para a Saúde das Pessoas Idosas. Direção Geral da Saúde. 2004.

20 Ferry M, Alix E. A nutrição na pessoa idosa – Aspectos fundamentais, clínicos e psicossociais. 2nd. ed. Lusociência, Loures. 2002.

6 Evaluation of indoor air quality and its importance for health and wellness promotion in the older adult

Ana Ferreira, António Loureiro, and Silvia Seco

Introduction

Environmental issues should deserve our full attention, because of the multitude of factors that contribute to our well-being and quality of life. These factors are the ones that occupy the top place, not only for the influence they have on our daily lives, but also because they condition our future. One of these issues is the quality of the air that surrounds us[1].

Air quality is a term commonly used to translate the degree of breathable air pollution, which is caused by a mixture of chemicals that are released into the air or result from chemical reactions that alter the natural constitution of the atmosphere. This change has negative repercussions on public health and well-being of the population but also has a detrimental influence on the fauna, flora, and material heritage[2].

Currently, there is an increasing concern with the problem of indoor air quality (IAQ) motivated by the increase of the permanence of the population in indoor environments, such as home, office, school, centers and nursing homes, commercial or administrative public places, among others. This is particularly relevant in urban populations, where it is estimated that 80–90% of their time is spent indoors and therefore more exposed to indoor air pollution than outdoor air pollution[3,4]. The good quality of the air we breathe is considered a basic requirement for human health and well-being[5]. The study of IAQ is essential in places where there are older adult, as they constitute a vulnerable risk group[6], which stays indoors an average of 19–20 hours[7]. This age group is exposed to a concentration of pollutants inside that is, sometimes, higher than outside[8].

DOI: 10.4324/9781003215271-6

The interior environment of buildings is contaminated by substances that result from the day-to-day use of these spaces or from materials in buildings. Depending on their characteristics and concentration, these substances can have an effect on the well-being of occupants, ranging from a mild feeling of discomfort to ultimately causing serious illness.

Several studies on air quality and their health implications have been conducted in order to evaluate the relationship between pollution indices and adverse health effects, making this theme increasingly pertinent[9]. Adverse health effects from inhalation of airborne pollutants may be immediate or felt some years later or over a long period of exposure. In order to maintain a suitable environment for the permanence of the occupants it is necessary to eliminate the harmful substances[10]. Table 6.1 shows some pollutants that can be found inside buildings and their main health effects.

Over the past decade, the onset of respiratory infections has often been associated with indoor air pollution, and the World Health Organization (WHO) has highlighted asthma, obstructive pulmonary disease, and lung cancer as some health problems that have arisen from a poor IAQ. Air pollution is a public health problem and the most common pollutants in the atmosphere, man being primarily responsible for their emission, are particulate matter (namely $PM_{2.5}$ and PM_{10}), carbon monoxide (CO), dioxide (CO_2), formaldehyde (CH_2O), and volatile organic compounds (VOCs). WHO highlights airborne particles, nitrogen dioxide, and tropospheric ozone as the most harmful air pollutants[11–13].

Carbon dioxide is a colorless, odorless, and non-flammable gas generated inside buildings, mainly through human metabolism[14]. Prolonged exposure to CO_2 can produce central nervous system effects such as headaches, dizziness, and visual problems. The concentration of CO_2 inside buildings is a great indicator of the ventilation rate of spaces[15].

Carbon monoxide is a colorless, odorless, extremely toxic, and suffocating gas that results from incomplete combustion of fossil fuels (wood, coal, oil, and gasoline). This pollutant is present when combustion gases are not properly vented to the outside of the building[14]. CO can cause symptoms such as dizziness, headache, nausea, ringing in the ears, heart palpitation, and irregular breathing, and in high concentrations of inhalation, this gas can be fatal[15].

Formaldehyde is a colorless gas that is flammable at room temperature, has an intense odor and is therefore easily detected by humans. In older adult institutions there may be uncontrolled emission of this pollutant from building or furniture materials and from the use of

Table 6.1 Effects of environmental pollutants on health

Environmental pollutants	Major health effects
Carbon monoxide – CO	Carboxyhemoglobinemia, headache, dizziness, tiredness, dizziness, drowsiness, reduced hearing and smell, impaired memory, decreased visual perception, decreased working ability, decreased manual dexterity, favors the deposition of cholesterol in the artery walls.
Carbon dioxide – CO_2	Asthma, whooping cough, breathing difficulties, headaches, tiredness, eye and throat irritation, central nervous system, and cardiovascular effects.
Volatile organic compounds – VOCs	Eye, nose, and throat irritation, allergies, nausea, leukemia, skin and lung cancer, headaches, fatigue, dizziness, kidney and liver effects, loss of balance, and infertility.
Ozone – O_3	Breathing problems, eye irritation, headache, changes in alertness and action, pulmonary edema if prolonged or repeated exposure, asthmatic and allergic reactions, dry mouth and throat, chest and cough pressure, bronchial inflammation, nose, and throat.
Formaldehyde – CH_2O	Burning sensation in the eyes, nose and throat, cough, tiredness, headache, abdominal pain, dizziness, anxiety, thirst, diarrhea, vomiting, nausea, disorders of sleep (drowsiness or insomnia), recent or past loss of concentration and memory, breathing difficulties, itching, and allergic reactions.
Asbestos	Breathing difficulties, lung tissue injury (Asbestosis), lung cancer, pleura (Mesothelioma), or peritoneum cancer.
Radon	It affects the bronchi, pulmonary alveoli and increases the risk of lung cancer.
Heavy metals	Behavioral (e.g., more aggressive), developmental (e.g., delayed physical development and shorter stature) and neurological system changes (e.g., mental retardation, cognitive difficulties including attention problems, lack of vocabulary and grammatical difficulties).
Sulfur dioxide – SO_2	Eye and respiratory tract irritation, asthma attacks, migraines, and headache.
Nitrogen oxides – Nox	Reversible or irreversible lesions in the lung bronchi and alveoli, pulmonary edema, chronic bronchitis, emphysema, eye and throat irritation, cough, and tiredness.
Particles	Nasal irritation, cough, bronchitis, asthma, and breathing difficulties.
Tobacco environment smoke	Mucosal irritation, chronic and acute effects on the respiratory tract, cardiovascular effects, and cancer.

non-exhaust equipment (gas stoves). According to WHO, these may cause burning in the eyes and throat, nausea, respiratory irritation, and asthmatic reactions. Studies indicate that formaldehyde may be carcinogenic to humans in the nasopharynx[14].

The suspended particles are in the form of fumes or dust and are released from various types of primary (combustion, industrial processes) and secondary (photo-oxidation products) sources. The particles can have various dimensions, being classified as PM_{10} (coarse particles) and $PM_{2.5}$ (fine particles). Particles are defined as "inhalable" if their aerodynamic diameter is below 10 μm. Exposure related effects include inflammatory airway reactions, adverse effects on the cardiovascular system, increased lung disease and, possibly, lung cancer[16,17].

Nanoparticles can be of natural origin (forest fires, marine pollution), unintentional anthropogenic origin (industrial pollution, indoor pollution), and intentional (industrial or laboratory scale nanoparticles). Humans may be exposed to these pollutants through inhalation, ingestion, or dermal contact, and the respiratory tract is the main pathway for nanoparticles to enter the body. Although studies on health effects are still insufficient, nanoparticles are expected to play an important role in the development of cardiovascular, respiratory, and central nervous system pathologies[18,19].

Sick Building Syndrome (SED) is a term used to describe situations of occupational discomfort and/or acute health problems reported by occupants, which may be related to staying inside some buildings. WHO has defined SED as a set of symptoms: headache, fatigue, lethargy, itching and burning eyes, nose and throat irritation, skin abnormalities, and poor concentration[20]. According to this organization, 20% of building occupants complain of physical problems when entering a building and that after leaving the building the symptoms gradually disappear or are alleviated[21]. Taking SED into account, we can see that ventilation is critical, as it is the process by which fresh air is intentionally supplied and stale air is removed. This process can be performed naturally or mechanically[22,23].

According to WHO, indoor air pollution is the eighth most important risk factor, accounting for 2.7% of the world's disease cases[11]. In Portugal, within the scope of the IAQ, diplomas have emerged that reflect the implementation of practical measures in defense of public health, regarding to IAQ. The need to reconcile energy efficiency with comfort and health promotion in indoor spaces has led to the development of the National Energy Certification System and IAQ in buildings, called ECS – Energy Certification System.

Existing ECS legal texts partially transposing Directive n.° 2010/31/EU on Energy Performance of Buildings, the European Parliament and the Council of 19 May are:

- Decree Law n.° 118/2013, of 20 August – aims to ensure and promote the improvement of energy performance of buildings through the ECS, which integrates the Energy Performance Regulation of Housing Buildings (EPR) and the Energy Performance Regulation of Commerce and Services Buildings (ERCS).
- Ordinance n.° 353-A/2013 of 4 December – establishes the minimum values of fresh air flow per space, as well as the protection thresholds and reference conditions for indoor air pollutants of new commercial and service buildings, subject to major and existing intervention and the evaluation methodology.

The Decree-Law n.° 118/2013 of 20 August has as its main objectives improvement of the overall energy efficiency of buildings, to impose efficiency rules on HVAC systems to improve their effective energy performance, to ensure the means to maintain a good IAQ and to inspect regularly the HVAC maintenance practices as a condition for energy efficiency and the IAQ.

In 2009, a Technical Note was published that sets out the methodology for auditing the IAQ. For Temperature (T°) and Relative Humidity (RU) the reference are the values established in the General Regulation of Hygiene and Safety at Work in Commercial Establishments, Offices and Services approved by Decree-Law n.° 243/86 of August 20[24-27].

The present work aimed to evaluate indoor and outdoor air quality, namely CO_2, CO, CH_2O, $PM_{2.5}$, PM_{10}, nanoparticles, T°, and Hr, in a day care center and also to verify the prevalence of symptoms and pathologies of the older adult. This research aimed to contribute to the knowledge of the problem of IAQ in buildings, particularly in the day care centers of the older adult, identify some of the health effects of pollutants, resulting from exposure to poor IAQ, as well as implement preventive measures in order to safeguard the health of the older adult who benefit from these institutions.

Material and methods

The target population consisted of 18 older adult from the day center under study, as well as the interior space (living room and dining room) and exterior space. The type of sampling was not probabilistic, accidental technique or for convenience. The type of study was observational level II, prospective in nature.

In order to evaluate IAQ, the following parameters were measured: CO_2, CO, $PM_{2.5}$, PM_{10}, nanoparticles, CH_2O, T°, and Hr. Also outside measurements were made for all the parameters mentioned above, except for formaldehyde. Measurements were taken from January to March, 2018 in two day care center locations: the living room and dining room. At each site, several measurements were taken throughout the day, namely at 9am, 12pm, and 4pm. Outside, the measurement was at 11am. Air quality measurements were performed on specific, portable, real-time reading equipment and were properly calibrated before taking measurements. The CO_2, CO, T°, and Hr were evaluated by Q. Track Plus IAQ Monitor, TSI model 8552/8554, with electrochemical cell. The $PM_{2.5}$ and PM_{10} measurements were performed using the Particles Counters, Lighthouse brand, Handheld model 3016 IAQ. The CH_2O was evaluated with the PPM Formaldemeter, htv model. Finally, the nanoparticles were evaluated with the P-Track equipment, brand TSI, model 8525.

IQA measurements were performed during the normal working hours of the day center, and the equipment was placed in the most central position of each space evaluated and approximately at the airway height of the older adult, in the sitting position.

Taking into account the legal standard, 2250 mg/m³ (1250 ppm) was considered as a reference for CO_2 protection thresholds, for CO, 10.0 mg/m³ (9 ppm), for $PM_{2.5}$, 25 µg/m³, for PM_{10}, 50 µg/m³ and for CH_2O, 0.01 mg/m³ (0.08 ppm). The reference ambient comfort conditions for T° C shall be between 18 and 22°C while Hr should be between 50% and 70%[24-27].

A questionnaire was administered to the older adult in order to verify their perception of IAQ, as well as the presence of symptoms and pathologies.

IBM SPSS Statistic software, version 25.0 was used to perform the statistical treatment of the collected data. The statistical tests applied were: Wilcoxon, Mann–Whitney, Kruskal–Wallis, Pearson Correlation and Spearman's Rho. For statistical inference we considered a confidence level of 95% for a random error of 5% or less.

Regarding the compliance to ethical standards in the scientific research, the participation of respondents in the study went through a phase of clarification of the objectives of the study, where the older adults were free to participate. The anonymity and confidentiality of the collected data were guaranteed.

Results

The study sample comprised the evaluation of IAQ (living room and dining room) and the evaluation of outdoor air quality near the day center.

Table 6.2 shows the values obtained for the pollutants studied.

According to the results obtained in Table 6.2, we found that there were statistically significant differences between the parameters CO_2, $T°$, Hr and nanoparticles, and the adopted environments (p-value < 0.05).

Through the analysis of the evaluated average values, we verified that the parameters $PM_{2.5}$, PM_{10}, CO_2, $T°$, and nanoparticles were higher inside the evaluated day center when compared to the outside environment. In the opposite sense, the parameters Hr and CO presented, on average, higher values in the outdoor environment.

Then, the average concentration of the environmental parameters, the living room and the day room refectory were evaluated (Table 6.3).

It was possible to verify that the average values of all the evaluated parameters were within the legally established protection threshold value, with the exception of $PM_{2.5}$ and PM_{10}.

Relating the average values of the studied parameters with the interior spaces evaluated in the day center, it was found that only statistically significant differences occurred for the meteorological variable $T°$, which was higher in the living room space when compared to the space refectory.

Table 6.2 Average concentration of environmental parameters

| | Space | | | |
| | inside | | Outside | |
	Average	Standard deviation	Average	Standard deviation
$PM_{2.5}$	38.25	17.76	33.28	25.85
PM_{10}	81.15	42.26	53.79	36.09
CO_2	1147.63	583.05	245.00	11.85
CO	2.48	0.42	2.60	0.66
Temperature	17.67	1.80	10.24	2.14
Relative humidity	64.36	8.01	77.46	13.34
Nanoparticles	610,556	81,773	12,344	10,857

Test: Mann–Whitney.

Table 6.3 Average concentration of environmental parameters by interior space evaluated

		Measurement location			
		Living room	Refectory	Total	p-value
$PM_{2.5}$	Average	36.64	39.87	38.25	0.694
	Standard deviation	16.58	19.30	17.76	
PM_{10}	Average	80.38	81.93	81.15	0.756
	Standard deviation	38.61	46.98	42.26	
CO_2	Average	1298.73	996.53	1147.63	0.171
	Standard deviation	661.26	466.91	583.05	
CO	Average	2.42	2.55	2.48	0.557
	Standard deviation	0.33	0.50	0.42	
CH_2O	Average	0.0007	<0.0001	0.0003	0.317
	Standard deviation	0.00258	0.00000	0.00183	
Temperature	Average	18.59	16.75	17.67	0.006
	Standard deviation	1.92	1.09	1.80	
Relative humidity	Average	61.64	67.09	64.36	0.110
	Standard deviation	6.85	8.36	8.01	
Nanoparticles	Average	41,689	80,422	61,055	0.468
	Standard deviation	15,451	113,176	81,772	

Regarding the analysis of the remaining parameters evaluated, by space, we found that, on average, the values were higher in the cafeteria when compared to the social room for the parameters $PM_{2.5}$, PM_{10}, CO, Hr, and nanoparticles. As for the CO_2 and CH2O parameters, these were higher in the social room, and in the case of CO_2, the value found was higher than the protection threshold value (1250 ppm).

Table 6.4 presents the analyzed parameters, as a function of the measurement time.

Data analysis shows that all parameters increased significantly throughout the day (*p*-value <0.05) except CO and CH_2O. It can be observed that PM_{10} and CO_2 were the pollutants that increased the most during the day, as well as the temperature. The measurements taken at 9h, 12h, and 16h were indoors, while the measurements made at 11h were outdoors.

Table 6.4 Average pollutant concentration, temperature, and relative humidity, depending on the time of measurement for indoor and outdoor

		Average	Standard deviation	Confidence interval – 95%	
				Inferior limit	Upper limit
$PM_{2.5}$	9.00h	28.69	14.85	18.01	39.31
	11.00h	33.28	25.85	1.18	65.37
	12.00h	34.00	16.44	22.24	45.76
	16.00h	52.07	13.83	42.18	61.96
	Total	37.54	18.72	31.11	43.97
PM_{10}	9.00h	50.14	19.65	36.08	64.20
	11.00h	53.79	36.09	8.98	98.61
	12.00h	72.69	35.83	47.05	98.32
	16.00h	120.64	34.71	95.81	145.46
	Total	77.25	42.08	62.79	91.70
CO_2	9.00h	546.40	145.52	442.30	650.50
	11.00h	245.00	11.85	230.28	259.72
	12.00h	1245.80	415.05	948.89	1542.71
	16.00h	1650.70	456.51	1324.13	1977.27
	Total	1018.69	626.64	803.43	1233.94
CO	9.00h	2.34	0.28	2.14	2.54
	11.00h	2.60	0.66	1.78	3.42
	12.00h	2.48	0.40	2.19	2.77
	16.00h	2.63	0.53	2.25	3.01
	Total	2.50	0.45	2.34	2.66
CH_2O	9.00h	0.0010	0.00316	−0.0013	0.0033
	11.00h	–	–	–	–
	12.00h	0.0000	0.00000	0.0000	0.0000
	16.00h	0.0000	0.00000	0.0000	0.0000
	Total	0.0003	0.00183	−0.0003	0.0010
Temperature	9.00h	16.16	1.14	15.34	16.98
	11.00h	10.24	2.14	7.58	12.90
	12.00h	18.84	1.81	17.54	20.13
	16.00h	18.00	1.30	17.07	18.93
	Total	16.61	3.20	15.51	17.71
Relative humidity	9.00h	59.16	5.76	55.03	63.28
	11.00h	77.46	13.34	60.89	94.03
	12.00h	64.06	8.58	57.92	70.20
	16.00h	69.87	5.98	65.59	74.15
	Total	66.23	9.86	62.85	
Nanoparticles	9.00h	41,209	17,276	28,850	53,567
	11.00h	12,343	10,857	−1137	25,825
	12.00h	98,230	137,055	186	196,273
	16.00h	43,729	12,538	34,760	52,698
	Total	54,097	77,566	27,452	80,742

Test: Kruskal–Wallis.

Table 6.5 Relationship between pollutants and temperature and relative humidity

		Temperature	Humidity	$PM_{2.5}$	PM_{10}	CO_2
Temperature	r	1	−0.048	0.048	0.191	**0.561**
	p		0.799	0.801	0.313	0.001
Relative humidity	r		1	0.154	0.314	**0.552**
	p			0.415	0.091	0.002
$PM_{2.5}$	r			1	**0.908**	0.372
	p				0.000	0.043
PM_{10}	r				1	**0.553**
	p					0.002
CO_2	r					1
	p					
CO	r					
	p					

Test: Pearson correlation.

Legend: r = Pearson correlation; p = p-value.

Then, the variation of atmospheric pollutants as a function of $T°$ and Hr of air in the interior spaces was evaluated.

As we can see through the analysis of Table 6.5, the estimated values of $T°$ correlated positively and significantly with the values of CO_2 (p-value < 0.05). It was possible to verify that the $T°$ was higher in places where the CO_2 levels were also higher. Regarding the Hr, there was a positive correlation with the atmospheric parameters CO_2 and CO (p-value < 0.05). It was also noticed that the places where the highest values of Hr were registered were also those in which significantly higher values of the aforementioned parameters were detected.

Finally, through a questionnaire applied to the older adult, an analysis was made of symptoms/pathologies of day care users, as illustrated in Table 6.6.

From the applied questionnaire and analyzing the estimated results (Table 6.6), it was found that headache was the most prevalent symptom, having been reported by 15 elderly people, followed by pruritus (itching), burning or irritation in the eyes and dizziness, manifested by ten elderly people.

Discussion

This study aimed to evaluate IAQ in a day care center in central Portugal, where several indoor pollutants that could be a threat to occupants' health were measured. Studies indicate that daily

Table 6.6 Presence of symptoms/pathologies in the older adult day center

Symptoms/pathologies	n	% column
Asthma	3	16.7
Chronic bronchitis	3	16.7
Whistles (hisses in the chest)	3	16.7
Sneezing crisis	6	33.3
Pneumoconioses	0	0
Allergies (rhinitis)	1	5.6
Headaches	15	83.3
Itching, burning or eye irritation	10	55.6
Irritation, itching, skin dryness	2	11.1
Dizziness	10	55.6
Digestive problems	3	16.7
Breathing difficulties	4	22.2
Total	18 seniors	100.0

exposure to air pollution may be associated with decreased respiratory function[28].

After analyzing the results obtained, it was found that the CO pollutant is below the protection threshold value, thus not constituting a threat to the health of the older adult. This pollutant results from human activities, as in the case of incomplete combustion processes of organic materials such as wood[29], and in the living room, the stove was lit daily. Certain studies indicate that in locations using wood burning stoves, CO concentrations are generally close to 6.0 ppm[14,30].

CO_2 in the indoor air results from the biological metabolism of its occupants, so values tend to be higher where people stay longer. In the cafeteria, the CO_2 values are below the protection threshold, but, on the other hand, the living room showed values of this pollutant above the protection threshold. Several studies argue that CO_2 is an indicator of the quality of indoor air renewal, and when values exceed 1000.0 ppm, it is related to an insufficient air renewal rate[31]. Loureiro et al. (2015), found that CO_2 levels were higher in the late afternoon[14]. Through the measurements we observed, in fact, the CO_2 values were higher at the end of the day compared to the early morning. Measurements of this pollutant performed at 9 am in the living room ranged from 400 ppm to 745 ppm, while at the end of the day the values were between 1520 ppm and 2438 ppm, with the protection threshold of this pollutant according to Ordinance n.° 353-A/2013, being 1250 ppm. Most likely the increase in CO_2 concentration was influenced by the absence of aeration. The living room windows were always closed (including before arrival and after the older adult left), aggravated by the fact that they have a quantity of decorative objects hanging on the windows, as well as on the sill, which makes them difficult to open.

Jesus et al. (2008) in their study reported that exposure to formaldehyde is likely to cause nasopharyngeal cancer[32]. In the present study, the average CH_2O values did not exceed the legally established protection threshold (0.08 ppm) and, as such, did not present a health hazard to day-care occupants[33].

Regarding the average concentrations of $PM_{2.5}$ and PM_{10}, several studies have been conducted relating PM exposure and increased hospitalization due to lung diseases[34]. The values obtained were found to exceed the protection threshold legally established in Ordinance 353-A/2013, 25 µg/m^3 and 50 µg/m^3, respectively. The increase in average particle concentration throughout the day, both in the living room and in the cafeteria, was notable. As mentioned above, the living room of the day center under study was equipped with wood-fired heating, which according to Loureiro et al. (2015), it is one of the factors that provides the increase of particles. Also the fact that there is a national road near the day center that can influence airborne particulate concentrations at times when the main door was open for people to enter/exit, as car traffic is one of the main sources emission of pollutants. In the study, on IAQ, Ferreira et al. (2014) mentioned that another probable cause for the high concentration of PM_{10} could be the presence of large amounts of paper, which, in the case of the living room, is present in the decorative objects on the walls and cabinets[16]. On the other hand, Buczynska et al. (2014) argues that in winter it is natural that there will be an increase in pollutants in the environment, since the cold air mass that remains close to the ground retains them. These results highlight the importance of regular control of $PM_{2.5}$ and PM_{10} concentrations within day centers, as they may aggravate or promote the onset of chronic respiratory diseases[34].

In the social room, the average nanoparticle value was 41,689 particles/cm^3 and in the cafeteria 80,422 particles/cm^3. These values, as well as other pollutants, may be related to the proximity to the kitchen, both in the living room and in the cafeteria[35]. The cooking process may release particulate matter, particularly in roasts, fried and grilled food[36]. Although there are no protection threshold values yet, studies have been conducted reporting that this pollutant may cause adverse health effects. According to Martins et al. (2015), nanoparticles can be harmful to the brain, causing Parkinson's or Alzheimer's diseases, and effect the lungs causing asthma or bronchitis. Also at the circulatory system and heart level, various problems can arise such as vasoconstriction, hypertension and arrhythmia or heart disease. Nanoparticles are likely to cause dermatitis and urticaria and may also cause colon cancer at the gastrointestinal system level[37].

$T°$ and Hr are also very important factors, contributing to the development/propagation of microorganisms, which may influence the health of the older adult. According to the General Regulation of Hygiene and Safety at Work in Commercial Establishments, Offices and Services approved by Decree-Law n.° 243/86 of 20 August, the temperature must be between 18 and 22°C. Hr values should be between 50 and 70%. The living room presented $T°$ and Hr values within the protection threshold, 18.6°C and 61.6%, respectively. On the other hand, in the cafeteria the temperature was slightly below the recommended 16.7°C, and Hr was within the established limit, 67%. The cafeteria was used only 3 times a day (breakfast, lunch, and snack) and as such the low temperature may be justified by the lack of occupants as well as the poor thermal insulation of the windows. Although Hr values were within the normal range, it is important to point out that both in the living room and in the cafeteria, the presence of mold on the ceiling and walls was remarkable, which is a source of microorganisms. The development of fungi and molds can cause various health problems for the older adult, such as respiratory infections, asthma, allergies, cough, among others[38].

The studied day center is located near the village center, with a national road 50 meters away. However, given that space ventilation was not promoted, sources of contamination are expected to be inside[4], particularly on decorative objects, on the heating system and occupants[39]. Despite being winter at the time of measurements, the spaces should still be aerated frequently, as Mendes et al. (2015) reports, given that it is a practice that can dramatically decrease the number of pollutants inside[40]. In order to avoid low indoor temperatures, ceilings, walls, and windows should be well insulated, thus maintaining natural ventilation whenever possible[41].

Finally, from the questionnaire applied to the older adult regarding the presence of symptoms/pathologies, it was found that headache was the most prevalent symptom (15 older adults). Also itching, burning or irritation in the eyes and dizziness were quite common symptoms in the older adult under study, each of these symptoms manifesting in 10 older adults. Several studies point to the fact that exposure to chemical pollutants promotes the development of various pathologies[16]. In order to avoid the presence of symptoms/pathologies caused by IAQ, outdoor leisure activities should be promoted whenever the health condition of the older adult allows it[42].

Conclusions

IQA monitoring is essential for defining an indoor approach and control strategies to eliminate or mitigate indoor environmental problems in order to achieve a minimally acceptable IAQ. We must not forget that, according to various studies, the indoor air pollution level can reach two to five times, occasionally 100 times, higher than the outdoor air pollution level[2,43-45].

With the results obtained in this study, we can conclude that it is necessary to take measures to improve the IAQ, since there were atmospheric pollutants, such as CO_2 (in the living room) and $PM_{2.5}$ and PM_{10} (in the living room and in the cafeteria) whose concentration was above that of the protection limit. Thus, it is essential that institutions carry out continuous monitoring in order not to expose the older adult to risk situations. The importance of improving air renovation systems is also emphasized in order to make air renovation more efficient and effective, choosing whenever possible natural ventilation, such as simply opening windows frequently.

Living rooms, which are considered the most sensitive areas, should be ventilated daily, even in winter for at least 15 minutes in the morning and 15 minutes in the afternoon. In addition, the composition of personal hygiene and cleaning products used should be analyzed to determine whether they contain compounds capable of causing risks to air quality and to the health of the older adult. It will also be necessary to analyze the possibility of adjusting the number of users per division, taking into account factors such as the area of space and the use percentage of the same.

Since CO_2 results essentially from the biological metabolism of living beings, it is recommended not to exceed the capacity of each living space under study, thus reducing the emissions of this pollutant, especially in spaces where the concentration was above the protection threshold value, or too close to that value. Another measure that can be considered is the use of certain plants, which have the capacity to absorb VOCs and help to eliminate chemicals present in the air, such as chlorophytum, comosum-aglaonema, spathiphyllum, dracaena, aloes, or creeper. This suggestion is made to help the air purification in spaces like living rooms[43,44].

Regarding nanoparticles, we considered that this theme should be discussed, given that the full consequences of exposure to this pollutant are not yet known, and that there is no legally established protection threshold. While $PM_{2.5}$ can be very harmful to people's health, nanoparticles can cause even more serious problems, given that they are smaller in size and can lodge in the human body more easily.

Through this study, it was possible to conclude that a good IAQ is fundamental for the well-being of the general population, but mainly for the older adult, considering that they spend most of their time inside buildings. Good IAQ should be achieved through the adoption of good practices regarding space ventilation and sanitation, as well as the correct implementation of building maintenance plans, such as: changes in occupant habits, replacement of materials used for decoration by easily washable ones, selection of environmentally friendly cleaners and ventilation of spaces whenever possible. IAQ should be a priority concern for the government and all health professionals, who should take action to preserve and improve air quality to prevent air pollutants from reaching concentrations that could endanger the health and well-being of the older adult.

Key points

- The indoor air pollution level can reach 2–5 times, occasionally 100 times, higher than the outdoor air pollution level.
- WHO highlights airborne particulate matter, nitrogen dioxide, and tropospheric ozone as the most harmful environmental pollutants for health.
- Exposure to particulate matter causes inflammatory airway reactions, adverse effects on the cardiovascular system and increased lung disease.
- Nanoparticles play an important role in the development of cardiovascular, respiratory, and central nervous system pathologies.
- The concentration of carbon dioxide inside buildings is a great indicator of the ventilation rate of spaces.

References

1 Lameiras H, Póvoas F. Qualidade do Ar – 1.a Edição. Coimbra: Comissão de Coordenação e Desenvolvimento Regional do Centro, 2003.

2 Déoux, S. Ecologia é a saúde. Divisão Editorial. s.l.: Instituto Piaget, 2001.

3 Costa, Ana Margarida, et al. Modelação de microscala da exposição a poluentes atmosféricos em áreas urbanas. X Congresso Nacional de Engenharia do Ambiente. CESAM, Departamento de Ambiente e Ordenamento, Universidade de Aveiro, Portugal: s.n., 2009.

4 Klepeis NE, et al. The national human activity pattern survey (NHAPS): A resource for assessing exposure to environmental pollutants. J Expo Anal Environ Epidemiol. 2001;11(3):231–52.

5 Almeida M, Lopes I, Nunes C. Caracterização da qualidade do ar interior em Portugal – Estudo HabitAR. Rev Port Imunoalergologia. 2010;18(1)21–38.

6   Infante A, Amaral MA. Análise da qualidade ambiente interior em infantários e lares de idosos. Dissertação de Mestrado em Engenharia de Construção e Reabilitação, Escola Superior de Tecnologia e Gestão de Viseu; 2016, pp. 5–36.

7   Nogueira S, Sobreira C, Aelenei D, Viegas J. Contribuição para o conhecimento da qualidade do ar interior em Lares de Idosos: Determinação do teror de CO_2 e de taxas de ventilação. Conferência Internacional sobre Envelhecimento – CISE 2013, 22 Novembro, Lisboa, Portugal. 2013, pp. 91–101.

8   Ferreira A, Cardoso M. Qualidade do ar e saúde em escolas localizadas em freguesias predominantemente urbanas, rurais e mediamente urbanas. Revista Brasileira de Geografia Médica e da Saúde. 2013;9(17)95–115.

9   Gioda A, Neto FR. Considerações sobre estudos de ambientes industriais e não industriais no Brasil: uma abordagem comparativa. 2003, pp. 1389–97.

10 Massa A. Auditoria à Qualidade do Ar Interior nos edifícios da Universidade do Minho em Azurém. s.l.: Escola de Engenharia da Universidade do Minho, 2010.

11 Pinto M, Rebelo A, Santos J, Vieira M. Avaliação da Qualidade do Ar Interior em Centros de Dia para Idosos. In: Occupational safety and hygiene: SHO 2012. 2010. p. 351–3.

12 Borrego C., et al. A Saúde e o Ar que respiramos – um caso de estudo em Portugal. Lisboa: Fundação Calouste Gulbenkian, 2008.

13 Gomes, João Pereira. Poluição Atmosférica – Um manual universitário. Porto: Publindústria, 2001.

14 Loureiro A, Ferreira A, Figueiredo J, Simões H. Qualidade do Ar Interior em Lares de Idosos e a Exposição Ocupacional aos Poluentes Atmosféricos. Dissertação de Mestrado em Segurança e Saúde do Trabalho, Escola Superior de Tecnologia da Saúde de Coimbra; 2015. Available fromhttp://hdl.handle.net/10400.26/14493.

15 Carmo AT, Prado RTA. Qualidade do Ar Interno. 1999.

16 Ferreira A, Cardoso M. Qualidade do Ar Interior em Escolas e Saúde das Crianças. Tese de Doutoramento em Ciências da Saúde, Faculdade de Medicina da Universidade de Coimbra; 2014. Available from http://hdl.handle.net/10316/26262.

17 Sobreira C, Viegas J, Aelenei D. Avaliação do desempenho da ventilação natural em lares de idosos. Dissertação de Mestrado em Engenharia Civil, Faculdade de Ciências e Tecnologia da Universidade Nova de Lisboa; 2015. Available from http://hdl.handle.net/10362/14745.

18 Matos L, Santos P, Barbosa F. As Nanopartículas em Ambientes Ocupacionais. 2011.

19 Pereira C, Gomes J, Albuquerque P. Contribuição para a caracterização da emissão de nanopartículas em processos de soldadura e avaliação de riscos decorrentes do processo. Dissertação de Mestrado em Engenharia Química e Biológica, Instituto Superior de Engenharia de Lisboa; 2014. Available from http://hdl.handle.net/10400.21/3308.

20 Bernardes Â, Martins N, Nunes T. Análise dos métodos de auditoria à qualidade do ar interior. Dissertação de Mestrado em Sistemas Energéticos Sustentáveis, Universidade de Aveiro; 2009. Available from http://hdl.handle.net/10773/663.

21 Amorim D, Silva S. Otimização das condições de ventilação natural em edifícios de serviço para assegurar a qualidade do ar interior sem consumos excessivos de energia. Dissertação de Mestrado em Engenharia Civil, Escola de Engenharia da Universidade do Minho; 2012. Available from http://hdl.handle.net/1822/29576.

22 Cerqueira F, Viegas J, Aelenei D. Avaliação das condições de ventilação de lares de idosos. Dissertação de Mestrado em Engenharia Civil, Faculdade de Ciências e Tecnologia da Universidade Nova de Lisboa; 2015. Available from http://hdl.handle.net/10362/15563.

23 Gonçalves M, Viegas J, Aelenei D. Estudo numérico do desempenho da ventilação num lar de idosos. Dissertação de Mestrado em Engenharia Civil, Universidade Nova de Lisboa; 2016. Available from http://hdl.handle.net/10362/19558.

24 Portaria n°. 353-A/2013 de 4 de Dezembro. Diário da República n°. 235 – I Série, s.l.: Ministério do Ambiente, Ordenamento do Território e Energia, da Saúde e da Solidariedade, Emprego e Segurança Social, 2013.

25 Decreto-Lei n°. 243/86 de 20 de Agosto. Diário da República n°. 190/1986 – I Série, Lisboa: Ministério do Trabalho e da Segurança Social, 1986.

26 Nota Técnica NT-ECS-02. Metodologia para auditorias periódicas da QAI em edifícios de serviços existentes no âmbito do RSECE. 2009.

27 Decreto-Lei n°. 118/2013 de 20 de Agosto. Diário da República n°. 159/2013 – I Série, Lisboa: Ministério da Economia e do Emprego, 2013.

28 Ferreira A, Cardoso S. Effects of indoor air quality on respiratory function of children in the 1st cycle of basic education of Coimbra. In: Arezes P, Baptista JS, Barroso MP, Carneiro P, Eds. *Occupational Safety and Hygiene II* (1st ed., p. 4), London: CRC Press, 2006.

29 Madureira J, Ferraz C, Mayan O. Impacte de uma grande linha de tráfego urbano na qualidade do ar e na saúde. Dissertação de Mestrado em Engenharia do Ambiente, Faculdade de Engenharia da Universidade do Porto; 2005. Available from https://hdl.handle.net/10216/11025.

30 Maio S, Sarno G, Baldacci S, I Annesi-Maesano GV. Air quality of nursing homes and its effect on the lung health of elderly residents. Expert Rev Respir Med. 2017;9(6):671–3. doi:10.1586/17476348.2015.1105742

31 Ginja J, Borrego C, Coutinho M, Nunes C. Qualidade do ar interior nas habitações Portuguesas:10.

32 Jesus L, Andrade I, Pocinho M, Girão A. Exposição Ocupacional ao Formaldeído, COV e Partículas: Impacto na Saúde Humana. 2008.

33 Qualidade do Ar em Espaços Interiores Um Guia Técnico [Internet]. Agência Portuguesa do Ambiente. 2009. p. 56. Available from: https://www.apambiente.pt/_zdata/Divulgacao/Publicacoe s/Guias e Manuais/manual QArInt_standard.pdf

34 Buczynska AJ, Krata A, Grieken R Van, Brown A, Polezer G, Wael K De, et al. Composition of $PM_{2.5}$ and PM_1 on high and low pollution event days and its relation to indoor air quality in a home for the elderly. Sci Total Environ. 2014;490:134–43.

35 Almeida-silva M, Wolterbeek HT, Almeida SM. Elderly exposure to indoor air pollutants. Atmos Environ. 2014;85:54–63.

36 Coentro S, Almeida S, Ferreira F. Qualidade do Ar Interior em habitações: Fontes emissoras de poluentes. Dissertação de Mestrado em Engenharia do Ambiente, Faculdade de Ciências e Tecnologia da Universidade Nova de Lisboa; 2015.

37 Martins L, Lopes Á. Toxicologia de nanomateriais. Instituto Superior de Ciências da Saúde Egas Moniz; 2015. Available from http://hdl.handle.net/10400.26/10918.

38 Brochado J, Barreira E, Almeida R. Desenvolvimento de bolores em edifícios de habitação – Análise de sensibilidade. Dissertação de Mestrado em Engenharia 32. Civil, Faculdade de Engenharia da Universidade do Porto; 2016. Available from https://hdl.handle.net/10216/85737.

39 Ferreira A, Cardoso S. Exploratory study of air quality in elementary schools, Coimbra, Portugal. Rev Saude Publica. 2013;47(6):1–9.

40 Mendes A, Bonassi S, Aguiar L, Pereira C, Neves P, Silva S, et al. Indoor air quality and thermal comfort in elderly care centers. Urban Clim. 2015;14:486–501.

41 Mendes A, Papoila A, Martins P, Bonassi S, Caires I, Palmeiro T, et al. The impact of indoor air quality and contaminants on respiratory health of older people living in long-term care residences in Porto. In: Age and ageing. 2016;45(1):136–42.

42 Ferreira A, Cardoso M. Qualidade do ar interno e saúde em escolas. J Bras Pneumol. 2014;40(3):259–68.

43 Sanguessuga, Marta. Síndroma dos Edifícios Doentes: Estudo da qualidade do ar interior e despiste da eventual existência de SED entre a população do edifício "E" de um estabelecimento de ensino superior. Disertação de Mestrado em Segurança e Higiene do Trabalho. s.l.: Escola Superior de Tecnologia da Saúde de Lisboa, Instituto Politécnico de Lisboa, Abril de 2012.

44 Strausz, M. Análise de um acidente fúngico na Biblioteca Central de Manguinhos: um caso de Síndroma do Edifício Doente. Revista Brasileira de Saúde Ocupacional. 2011;32(115):69–78.

45. European Environmental Agency. Environment and Health, EEA report N°. 10/2005; 2005.

7 Pharmacological treatment and the polymedicated older adult

Ana Paula Fonseca and Vera Galinha

Introduction

The increase in longevity and of the older population, together with the reduction in birth rates, has caused profound demographic changes in Portugal, similar to what has happened in the rest of Europe. In 2015, average life expectancy reached 77.4 years for men and 83.2 years for women, and people aged 65 and over represented 20.5% of the entire population resident in the country. Also, according to 2015 data, the rate of aging went from 27.5% in 1961 to 143.9% in 2015.[1]

According to the World Health Organization (WHO),[2] active aging is defined as the process of optimizing opportunities for health, participation and safety to improve quality of life as people age, as well as the process of developing and maintaining functional capacity, which contributes to the well-being of the older adult. However, if on the one hand, aging is the triumph of socioeconomic development and public health, on the other hand, it triggers a challenge of adaptation in society.[3]

To combine this cross-cutting issue with the various sectors of society, a project was designed to promote healthy aging through the implementation of an intervention program based on comprehensive geriatric assessment (in Portuguese, Abordagem Geriátrica Ampla – AGA),[4] incorporating regional and academic endogenous resources. The proposed AGA model is based on an individual holistic model, supported by a multidisciplinary assessment protocol, from which the implemented intervention strategies, adjusted to the needs of each person, aim to prevent the frailty and functional, cognitive and social decline of the older adult. Intervention actions are focused on personalized exercise programs, nutritional education, cognitive stimulation,

DOI: 10.4324/9781003215271-7

third-party follow-up, therapeutic counseling and overall promotion of well-being.[4-6]

The issue of pharmacological medication in the older adult assumes particular importance, in the context of comorbidity in which aging commonly stems, causing major intrinsic challenges, such as the management of polymedication and the associated therapeutic complexity and adherence to therapy.

Polymedication in the older adult

Living longer means being more exposed to risks, such as vulnerability of health, physical and mental dependence, among others. Chronic noncommunicable diseases (cardiovascular diseases, respiratory diseases, cancer, diabetes *mellitus*, among others), mental and neurological disorders are some of the conditions that contribute to these comorbidities.[7] The treatment and management of these various chronic diseases affecting the older population means that polypharmacy has a special focus in this context, as multidrug administration over long periods is frequent.[8] Although it has no consensual definition, polypharmacy can be defined as the concomitant use of four or more medicines, if prescribed and/or self-medicated.[9]

In addition to medicines administered for the various chronic conditions, as indicated by a doctor, the older population self-medicate with a large number of non-prescribed medicines and dietary supplements, without any advice from a healthcare professional and without knowledge of the consequences that may result from their association with prescribed medicines.[10]

Adherence to therapy

Adherence to therapy is known to be a complex yet crucial element in obtaining the desired clinical and therapeutic results.[11] Patients who do not adhere to the therapy may present complications or the worsening of the pathologies, due to misuse of medication, triggering frequent hospitalization and economically heavier procedures for the health system. For an older patient, adherence to the prescribed therapy is crucial in order to obtain a positive result for their health.[12] However, it must be taken into account that along with advancing age, there is also a decrease in cognitive and functional abilities, which may result in greater difficulty in adhering to the prescribed therapy.[12,13]

Medication adherence is described as the process by which patients administer their medication as prescribed. The adherence process can be described in four steps: initiation, implementation, interruption and persistence.[14]

According to WHO, 50% of people with chronic diseases in developed countries are somehow non-compliant with drug therapies, and this percentage is higher in developing countries. Given this, we can say that non-adherence to therapy is now considered one of the biggest public health problems.[15]

The same organization (WHO) describes adherence as a multidimensional phenomenon, determined by the interaction of five groups of factors/dimensions: socioeconomic factors, factors related to the health system and equipment, factors related to the patient's condition, factors related to treatment and patient-related factors.[16] For each dimension, there are various possible reasons for non-adherence, ranging from complex therapeutic plans, difficulty in understanding medical prescriptions, patient dissatisfaction with health services, treatment of asymptomatic diseases, socioeconomic aspects and the beliefs of patients.[15] Several studies have shown that these determinants are central to adherence to therapy.

There are several strategies that can, and should, be adopted that have been shown to be effective in increasing adherence to therapy and consequently promote the achievement of quality clinical outcomes.[17] Individualized interventions, reminders of medication use, information on pharmacotherapy, self-monitoring, and qualified counseling, among others, are some of the measures that have been shown to be effective in increasing adherence to therapy and, consequently, to achieve positive clinical results.[18] The adoption of these measures is aimed at improving adherence to therapeutic medication which may bring benefits not only to the patient but also to health systems, as non-adherence has a very negative impact on health systems.

The therapeutic complexity

In the geriatric population, the evaluation of therapeutic complexity and the identification of its determinants is an increasingly necessary practice. The simplification of therapeutic regimens in this population improves treatment adherence, with benefits in medication adherence and consequently in therapeutic results, as well as in the quality of life of the older adult. Based on these facts the complexity of the therapeutic regimen has increasingly become a major concern for patients with chronic diseases and in particular in the geriatric population, as it can play a major role in non-adherence to the therapeutic regimen scheme.[19-21]

The complexity of the therapeutic regimen depends on several characteristics such as, number of medicines consumed, dosage forms, frequency of administration and additional instructions given by the doctor.[22] However, in literature there are several definitions of complexity of pharmacotherapy. In this context the *Medication Regimen Complexity Index (MCRI)* appeared, as the first specific and validated instrument, developed by George et al.,[22] in 2004, which aims to standardize the measurement of the complexity of pharmacotherapy. Years later, in 2007, the Índice de Complexidade da Farmacoterapia (ICFT) was issued, which is an adapted and validated version of the MCRI, in the Portuguese language, developed with the purpose of standardizing the concept of pharmacotherapy complexity, for clinical use as well as for research purposes.[23]

Complex treatment regimens are uncomfortable for both patients and physicians, not only because of non-adherence problems, but also due to the failure of therapeutic response or adverse drug reactions, as well as its effect upon the quality of life of the patients.

AGA@4life model and the therapeutic management of the older adult

Adherence management is described as the process of monitoring and supporting drug adherence by health systems, professionals, patients and their social networks. The purpose of this is to obtain the best use of prescription drugs to maximize the potential for benefit and minimize the risk of harm.[14]

Carers can play an extremely important role in overcoming barriers related to adherence to therapy, such as aid in drug administration, monitoring and psychological support.[19]

Accordingly, it is important to evaluate the adherence level of institutionalized older patients, as well as the factors that influence it, namely the complexity of pharmacotherapy, in order to outline future strategies to improve adherence.

The AGA@4life project provided a favorable ecosystem for the analysis of these issues by the application of two questionnaires, one for assessing adherence to therapy and another for assessing the complexity of the pharmacotherapeutic regimen. The questionnaire used to assess adherence to therapy consisted of three parts:

I Sociodemographic Characterization (age, gender, marital status, educational level, institutionalization time and the person responsible for preparing medication).
II Therapeutic Characterization (amount of daily medications and therapeutic regimen).
III Assessment of Adherence to Therapy, through the Treatment Adherence Measure (TAM) scale, consisting of seven questions to be answered on a scale of "always" to "never." The answers obtained are scored from 1 to 6, according to the following meaning: 1 – does not adhere fully; 2 – does not adhere; 3 – minimally adheres; 4 – partially adheres; 5 – mostly adheres; 6 – fully adheres). This scale was developed and validated for Portuguese by Delgado and Lima, in 2001, based on the questionnaire by Morisky et al.[24,25]

Regarding the evaluation of the complexity of the therapeutic regimen, the ICFT, the Portuguese version of the *Medication Regimen Complexity Index (MRCI)*[23] was used. This index is divided into three sections (A, B and C) which correspond respectively to information about the medication (section A), information on the frequency of dosage (section B) and additional information needed for specific medication (section C). Analyzing each patient individually, as well as the drugs they used, the different sections are then calculated and the sum results in an ICFT value.[23]

Conclusions

Polymedication and its associated complex therapeutic regimens are common features among the older population, as they have multiple comorbidities requiring the use of various medications to control or prevent them. Therefore, a more careful approach and careful monitoring of the pharmacotherapeutic profile of the older adult is essential, as well as the need to train health professionals, family members, the older adult and caregivers in managing the therapeutic regimen in order to derive their highest benefit.

A multidisciplinary approach based on an individual holistic model of the older adult, using an intervention plan adjusted to the needs of each person, can contribute to the improvement of care and to the reduction of common problems associated with the older adult such as frailty, functional, cognitive and social decline, as well as a reduction in hospitalization, and consequently, a reduction in health expenses.

Key points

- Increased population longevity is associated with the increase of chronic conditions and consequently the increase in polymedication.
- Prescribing potentially inappropriate medications increases the predisposition to adverse interactions and reactions.
- Adherence to therapy tends to be low in the polymedicated older adult.
- Pharmacotherapeutic complexity tends to be high due to the coexistence of several morbidities;
- Effective management of the treatment regimen increases adherence to therapy in institutionalized patients.

References

1 PORDATA. Base de Dados Portugal Contemporâneo. 2015.
2 World Health Organization. Ageing and health. 2018. http://www. who.int/news-room/fact-sheets/detail/ag.
3 Angeloni S, Borgonovi E. An ageing world and the challenges for a model of sustainable social change. J Manag Dev. 2016;35:464–85.
4 Solomon DH. Foreword. In: Osterweil D, Brummel-Smith K B. Comprehensive Geriatric Assessment. New York, NY: McGraw Hill. 2000.
5 Ong T. Ageing positively. J Prim Health Care. 2016;8:86.
6 Kogan AC, Wilber K, Mosqueda L. Person-centered care for older adults with chronic conditions and functional impairment: a systematic literature review. J Am Geriatr Soc. 2016;64(1):e1–7.
7 Grupo de trabalho Interministerial. Estratégia Nacional para o Envelhecimento ativo e saudável 2017-2025. Direção Geral da Saúde. Portugal. 2017.
8 Marengoni A, et al. Coexisting chronic conditions in the older population: variation by health indicators. Eur J Intern Med. 2016;31:29–34.
9 Rankin A, Cadogan CA, Patterson SM, Kerse N, Cardwell CR, Bradley MC, Ryan C, Hughes C. Interventions to improve the appropriate use of polypharmacy for older people. Cochrane Database Syst Rev. 2018;9:CD008165.
10 Amoako EP, Richardson-Campbell L, Kennedy-Malone L. Self-Medication with over-the-counter drugs among elderly adults. J Gerontol Nurs. 2004;29:10–5.
11 Roque Obreli-Neto P, de Oliveira Baldoni A, Molino Guidoni C, Bergamini D, de Carvalho Hernandes K, Toalhares da Luz R, et al. Métodos de avaliação de adesão à farmacoterapia Methods for estimating adherence to the pharmacotherapy. Rev Bras Farm. 2012;93(4):403–10.
12 Rocha CH, Oliveira AP, Ferreira, C, et al. Adesão à prescrição médica em idosos de Porto Alegre, RS. Ciênc. saúde coletiva [Internet]. 2008;13(Suppl):703–10.

13 Galvão C. O idoso polimedicado – Estratégias para melhorar a prescrição. Rev Port Med Geral e Fam. 2006;22(6):747–52.

14 Vrijens B, De Geest S, Hughes DA, Przemyslaw K, Demonceau J, Ruppar T, et al. A new taxonomy for describing and defining adherence to medications. Br J Clin Pharmacol. 2012;73(5):691–705.

15 WHO. Adherence to long-term therapies. 2003.

16 Kardas P, Lewek P, Matyjaszczyk M. Determinants of patient adherence: a review of systematic reviews. Front Pharmacol. 2013;4:91.

17 Neto PO. Fatores interferentes na taxa de adesão à farmacoterapia em idosos atendidos na rede pública de saúde do Município de Salto Grande – SP, Brasil. Rev Ciências. 2010;31(5790):229–33.

18 Obreli-Neto PR, Guidoni CM, de Oliveira Baldoni A, Pilger D, Cruciol-Souza JM, Gaeti-Franco WP, et al. Effect of a 36-month pharmaceutical care program on pharmacotherapy adherence in elderly diabetic and hypertensive patients. Int J Clin Pharm. 2011;33(4):642–9.

19 Jin J, Sklar GE, Min Sen Oh V, Chuen Li S. Factors affecting therapeutic compliance: a review from the patient's perspective. Ther Clin Risk Manag. 2008;4(1):269–286.

20 Marcum ZA, Gellad WF. Medication adherence to multidrug regimens. Clin Geriatr Med. 2012 May;28(2):287–300.

21 Elliott R. Impact of hospitalisation on the complexity of older patients' medication regimens and potential for regimen simplification. J Pharm Pract Res. 2011;41(1):21–5.

22 Johnson G, Yee-Teng P, Bailey MJ. Development and validation of the medication regimen complexity index. Ann Pharmacother. 2004;38:1369–76.

23 Melchiors AC, Correr CJ, Fernández-Llimos F. Translation and validation into Portuguese language of the medication regimen complexity index. Arq Bras Cardiol. 2007;89(4):210–8.

24 Delgado A, Lima ML. Contributo para a validação concorrente de uma medida de adesão aos tratamentos. Psicol saúde doenças. 2001;2(2):81–100.

25 Monterroso L, Pierdevara L, Joaquim N. Avaliação da adesão regime terapêutico dos utentes seguidos na consulta externa de psiquiatria do centro hospitalar barlavento algarvio. Revista Portuguesa de Enfermagem de Saúde Mental. 2012;7(2012):39–45.

8 The effect of auditory training in the older adult's lives

Carla Matos Silva, Carolina Fernandes, and Clara Rocha

Introduction

Population aging is an increasingly current reality worldwide and thus it is important to understand all the aspects involved in it, either at a social, economic level or at the level of health care.[1] Aging is defined as a set of transformations associated to the passage of years that bring psychological, physiological, and biological changes.[2]

With aging, several modifications appear at sensorial level, namely hearing loss associated to aging: presbycusis resulting from the sum of some extrinsic and intrinsic factors that will influence individuals' peripheral auditory system.[3] This type of hearing loss is a consequence of inner ear hair cells' degeneration that mainly affects the base zone of the cochlea. This means a progressive bilateral sensorineural type hearing loss that will influence the auditory perception of the individual and consequently influence his quality of life.[1,3]

As presbycusis is associated to aging, it tends to increase with aging.[2,4] According to Carvalho and Guarinello,[2] it is estimated that this decreasing of auditory acuity affects more than 60% of the population, hearing loss being the 4th most frequent problem found in the geriatric population.[5]

The auditory system is a keystone in the development of oral communication. The impairment of this system, at peripheral or central level, leads to an impaired capacity to maintain coherent speech, that is, there will be a consequent compromise at the level of acquisition and/or processing of the acoustic stimulus.[3]

The Central Auditory Processing (CAP) is responsible for the perceptive processing of auditory information in the Central Nervous System and for the neurobiological activity implied in its processing, involving the auditory pathways to the cortex that perform determined specific tasks on which the individual depends to interpret

DOI: 10.4324/9781003215271-8

verbal and non-verbal sounds.[6,7] Considering that the changes at the CAP level are characterized by the difficulty in interpreting the sound signal, even if the individual presents normal hearing, it is common that the Audiologist comes across the existence of an increased difficulty in the older population's speech perception, mainly in ambient noise, independently of the hearing loss degree.[1,8,9] According to Neves and Feitosa,[9] this increased difficulty is due to the influence of aging, not only at the peripheral auditory level, but also due to a deterioration at the level of the CAP as a consequence of the age-related modifications in the central areas of the nervous auditory system.

The capacity for processing auditory information requires an acute neurological coordination between all the structures of the auditory pathway. This information is received by both cerebral hemispheres in a dichotic way, that is, similar and at the same time so that the brain can search for standards and similarities in this information. In the presence of noise, there is an impairment of the received information mainly if the auditory stimuli (signal) come from one of the sides. Through inter-hemispheric communication, the missing signal in one side will be filled, assuring an intact reception. The behavioral tests used in the CAP evaluation provide difficult listening tasks in a controlled environment, thus identifying the impaired CAP capacities.[6,7]

Although many people have a normal auditory acuity (they detect the sounds within normal standards), they present difficulties interpreting the sounds, which may cause problems in language understanding.[9]

According to Bellis,[10] the CAP evaluation tests are classified in four different categories. We focus on the low redundancy monaural tests in which the extrinsic redundancy of the speech signal is decreased to evaluate the central processing function and the auditory closing of the information that encompasses attention and phonological representation. There are different types of low redundancy monaural tests, namely the filtered speech test, the speech test with noise, the compressed speech test, the compressed sentences test, the sentences test with ipsilateral competitive message and the pediatric test of speech intelligibility with ipsilateral competitive message.[10]

Gonçales and Cury[11] claim that the tests to evaluate the speech understanding in noise or reverberant situations should be part of the battery of tests on older adult in order to evaluate specific auditory functions such as memory, selective attention and information processing speed through the auditory pathway, which impact on speech understanding irrefutably interfering in older adult's communication abilities. Social isolation is one major consequence of this communication impairment leading to depressive states and to life quality degradation.[11]

In Portugal the CAP evaluation has been little valued due to, on one hand, the shortage of instruments for its evaluation in European Portuguese, and on the other hand, to the absence of scientific studies that would prove that the CAP evaluation and hearing training presents promising results even when we deal with the older population. Currently, the older adult auditory evaluation is restricted to the peripheral auditory system evaluation in order to implement auditory rehabilitation programs, neglecting the CAP evaluation, which, if included, would optimize the benefits of an auditory rehabilitation program. Thus, it is important to highlight the importance of the central auditory pathway study through auditory processing tests that will be fundamental to understand how aging can influence the different auditory abilities. The most used tests are: the filtered speech test, the speech test in noise and the sentences test with ipsilateral competitive message.[12-16]

Filtered speech test

The filtered speech test was developed by Ivey in 1969 and was one of the first low redundancy tests to be applied in clinical practice.[12] It is a monotonic test of acoustic signal discrimination, restricted in frequency, that evaluates the auditory capacities of auditory closing and discrimination. It also permits evaluation of the handling capacity of the intrinsic and extrinsic redundancies of language. In this test, the frequencies of the speech sounds are filtered in order to simulate an unintelligible or low understanding speech. When the individual has a normal CAP, he is able to perform the auditory closing, filling in the distorted or absent parts of the auditory signal, and thus recognizing the message.[12]

The normality criterion for this test corresponds to the proportion of correct answers equal or above 78%, being the performance of the second ear tested normally superior to the first.[13] In the preliminary study of Martins et al., the normality cut-off obtained for the Portuguese population was 77%.[14]

Speech in noise test

The main objective of this test is to measure the performance-intensity function comparing the recognition of speech in and out of a competitive noise environment. The patients with brainstem lesion tend to present many difficulties in recognizing speech in noise.[15]

In this test, monosyllables or disyllables are used from a phonetically balanced list, with an ipsilateral speech presentation and
with competitive noise (usually white noise), with a signal/noise
relation (SNR) between 0 and +10 dB. The speech is always presented at the same intensity, 40 dB above the auditory threshold,
measured previously with a simple tonal audiogram and the individual who is being evaluated is asked to repeat each word heard.
The result of this test is then compared with the result of the simple tonal audiogram.[16]

The normality reference criterion for the ability of auditory closing
in this test is above 70% correct answers for both ears.[16]

Sentences test with ipsilateral competitive message

The sentence test with competitive message has two versions: one is
intended for pediatric population and the other one for adult population.[17] The objective of this test is to understand the capacity of the
individual's auditory system to recognize verbal sounds in dichotic
and monotic listening. However, in the version applied to adults the
test is based on reading and in the one for children it is based on
pictures. Through this exercise of sentence recognition and in the
presence of several competitive noises, it is possible to observe the
individual's capacity to perform simple activities in his daily life in
noisy environments such as shopping centers, public transports or at
school.[17]

In the presence of abnormal results in the CAP evaluation tests,
an individual auditory training plan should be designed and implemented, aimed at stimulating the auditory pathway in order to
maximize the plasticity of the central nervous system. Thus it will
permit improvement of the perception of the auditory information
through formal and informal training in conflict situations which
will after enable greater comfort of communication even in adverse
environments.[8,9]

Auditory training dates back to the 6th century when bells were
used to stimulate the audition of deaf people.[18,19] In the beginning
of the 20th century, Goldstein and Forester carried out studies in
auditory training and concluded that people who received auditory
training had significant improvements in speech understanding
although these improvements were not seen at the auditory thresholds level.[18,19]

The objective of the current study was to evaluate the effect of the
auditory training on the older people's speech understanding.

Methodology

The current study enrolled 16 subjects aged between 65 and 91 years old, all community dwelling older adults. The sample was constituted of 9 female subjects (56.2%) and 7 male subjects (43.8%).

The tests used were the otoscopy, tympanogram and the Simple Tonal Audiogram in the frequencies of 500 Hz, 1000 Hz, 2000 Hz, 4000 Hz, and 8000 Hz. Posteriorly, all the subjects with light to moderate hearing loss underwent the CAP test, speech in noise test with a SNR of 10 dB and 15 dB.

In the speech in noise test, disyllables from a phonetically balanced list were used with the speech in ipsilateral presentation and competitive noise. The speech (signal) was presented with the same intensity – 50 dB above the medium tonal loss value previously measured with a simple tonal audiogram. The noise was presented at 10 dB or 15 dB below the signal. During testing the individual was asked to repeat each of the words heard.

All the individuals who had severe to profound grade hearing loss were excluded from the study as it was not possible to perform the speech test in noise, regardless of the signal/noise ratio, since the sound stimulus is presented at 50 dB HL above the medium tonal loss. Due to this fact, many older people were excluded from the study as they had severe to profound grade sensorineural deafness, which made it impossible to continue the application of the auditory training program. This observation illustrates the degradation of older adult's auditory health and the lack of investment in auditory rehabilitation programs, with serious implications in these individuals' quality of life.

After carrying out the peripheral and central evaluation of the auditory system, the formal auditory training started. The formal auditory training was constituted of 10 sessions during 5 weeks where the subjects were divided into two groups of 8 elements. Group 1 (G1) underwent an auditory training based on the speech in noise test and group 2 (G2) underwent the filtered speech test. This distribution was made according to the difficulties discovered during the evaluation of the speech in noise test. Those who revealed more difficulties in the speech in noise test were integrated into the G2.

Results

The audiometric curve highlights significant effects in the frequency with a decline from the frequency 500 Hz ($p<.001$ for both ears).

Before carrying out the auditory training, the medium tonal hearing loss (MTHL) for the right ear was of 32.50 dB (±10.39) and of 31.48 dB (±9.03) for the left ear. After the auditory training, the MTHL decreased to 32.2 dB (±10.59) for the right ear and to 31.25 dB (±9.9) for the left ear.

Relative to the results of the speech test in noise for the right ear before the training, we got 24.31% accuracy in the 10 dB SNR, 33.56% accuracy for the 15 dB SNR, with a total accuracy of 28.94%. After the auditory training, we verified an accuracy of 39.31% for the right ear in the 10 dB SNR, 46.13% in the 15 dB SNR and 43.38% in total.

As for the left ear, the results of the CAP test – speech in noise test before the training, were 31.13% accuracy in the 10 dB SNR, 35.13% accuracy in the 15 dB SNR and 33.06% accuracy in total. Similarly to the right ear, the percentage of successes also increased in the left ear in all the conditions of the test after the auditory training, where we noted 40.13% accuracy in the 10 dB SNR, 44.31% in the 15 dB SNR and 41.5% accuracy in total.

Through the comparison of the results of older adult's performance in the speech in noise test, pre and post auditory training, the accuracy increase in both ears was noticeable and statistically significant, independently of the SNR. Regarding the type of training, the G1 was more efficient than the G2.

Discussion/Conclusion

Comparing the results obtained before and after the auditory training, we verified significant improvements in the speech recognition test in noise in all the conditions of the test, in the 10 dB and 15 dB SNR and total in both ears. However, there were not significant variations in the auditory thresholds comparing the conditions before and after the auditory training.

The results of this preliminary study are similar to the ones presented by Beier et al.[20] This suggests that the auditory training must be performed to minimize the difficulties of speech understanding, mainly in noisy environments, in order to decrease the gaps in information processing and to strengthen the identification and discrimination of the sound patterns. Moreover, the re-education for the sound stimulation through activities that aim at re-introducing the sound stimuli will enable a change at the level of the older person's central auditory system morphology and physiology.[3,8,20,21]

Thus, technical hearing aids are not enough to solve hearing loss. The correct stimulation as well as the auditory training will bring a greater benefit and gain with the technical hearing aids and will minimize the impact of hearing loss associated to aging and improve older people's quality of life.[3]

In conclusion, the current study demonstrated benefits of auditory training interventions for improving the auditory processing, namely in the discrimination of speech in noise, thus minimizing the impact of hearing loss for older people. So, all the older adults with difficulties in speech understanding, especially in noisy environments that can compromise speech understanding, should be carefully evaluated and counseled about the benefits of auditory training. It should be noted that, according to some studies, the environment and all the auditory requirements which the individual will come across in his daily life will have a fundamental role in the preservation and reinforcement of the trained auditory abilities gained during the auditory training sessions.[22-24]

Key points

- With aging, hearing loss tends to increase, hampering speech understanding, mainly in noisy environments.
- The CAP evaluation should be part of a series of audiological exams for the older adult in order to evaluate not only the peripheral auditory system but also the central auditory system.
- The CAP evaluation permits guiding the older adult to auditory training programs.
- The auditory training will permit significant improvements in competitive messages minimizing the impacts of hearing loss in speech understanding.
- The accuracy of the CAP tests increases significantly after the auditory training.

References

1 Martin J S, Jerger JF. Some effects of aging on central auditory processing. Journal of Rehabilitation Research & Development. 2005;42(4):25–44.

2 Ruschel CV, Carvalho CR, Guarinello AC. The efficiency of an auditory rehabilitation program in elderly people with presbycusis and their family. Revista da Sociedade Brasileira de Fonoaudiologia. 2007;12(2):95–8.

3 Veras R, Mattos L. Audiologia do envelhecimento: revisão da literatura e perspetivas atuais. Revista Brasileira de Otorrinolaringologia. 2007;73(1):128–34.

4 Ng JH, Loke AY. Determinants of hearing-aid adoption and use among the elderly: a systematic review. International Journal of Audiology. 2015;54(5):291–300.

5 Buss LH, Graciolli LS, Rossi AG. Auditory processing in elderly: implications and solutions. Revista CEFAC. 2010;12(1):146–51.

6 ASHA. Central Auditory Processing: current status of research and implications for clinical practice. American Journal of Audiology. 1995;5(2):41–54.

7 ASHA. American Speech Language Hearing Association. (Central) Auditory Processing Disorders. Retrieved Março 4, 2011. http://www. asha.org/members/deskref-journals/deskref/default.

8 Cruz ACA, Andrade, NA, Gil D. A eficácia do treinamento auditivo formal em adultos com distúrbio do processamento auditivo (central). Revista CEFAC. 2013;15(6):1427–34.

9 Neves VT, Feitosa MA. Controversies or complexity in the relationship between temporal auditory processing and aging? Revista Brasileira de Otorrinolaringologia. 2003;69(2):242–9.

10 Bellis T. Assessment and Management of Central Auditory Processing Disorders in the Educational Setting: From Science to Practice (2nd ed.). San Diego, CA: Plural Publishing. 2001.

11 Gonçales AS, Cury MCL. Assessment of two central auditory tests in elderly patients without hearing complaints. Brazilian Journal of Otorhinolaryngology. 2011;77(1):24–32.

12 Bellis T. Assessment and Management of Central Auditory Processing Disorders in the Educational Setting: From Science to Practice. San Diego, CA: Singular Publishing. 1996.

13 Bellis T, Beck B. Central Auditory Processing in Clinical Practice. Retrieved Maio 13, 2015, from Audiology online: http://www.audiologyonline.com/articles/central-auditory-processing-in-clinical-1281.

14 Martins J, Alves M, Pereira C, Teixeira A. Bateria de Testes de Processamento Auditivo Central – Dados Normativos para a População adulta – Dados Preliminares. Porto: Poster apresentado no 60° Congresso Nacional da SPORL. 2013.

15 Rivabem K. Linguagem Escrita e Distúrbios do Processamento Auditivo Central: Uma Relação de Casualidade Contraditória. Dissertação apresentada à Universidade Tuiuti do Panamá para a obtenção do título de Mestre em Distúrbios da Comunicação, Curitiba. 2006.

16 Pereira L, Schochat E. Testes Auditivos Comportamentais para Avaliação do Processamento Auditivo Central. São Paulo: Pró-Fono. 2011.

17 Vellozo FF, Filha VAVS, Costa MJ, Biaggio EPV, Garcia MV. Teste de identificação de sentenças sintéticas com mensagem competitiva ipsilateral pediátrico: revisão narrativa sobre a sua aplicabilidade. Revista CEFAC. 2015;17(5):1604–16.

18 Musiek F. Auditory training and CAPD: a short history. The Hearing Journal. 2006;59(8):52.

19 Musiek F, Chermak G. Handbook of (Central) Auditory Processing Disorder. San Diego, CA: Plural Publishing Inc. 2007.

20 Beier LO, Pedroso F, Ferreira MIDC. Benefícios do treinamento auditivo em usuários de aparelho de amplificação sonora individual – revisão sistemática. Revista CEFAC. 2015;17(4):1327–32.

21 Kozlowski L, Wiemes GM, Magni C, Silva AL. A efectividade do treinamento auditivo na desordem do processamento auditivo central: estudo de caso. Revista Brasileira de ORL. 2004;70(3):427–32.

22 Pereira LD. Processamento auditivo. Temas em Desenvolvimento. 1993;2(11):7–14.

23 Schochat E, Carvalho LZ, Megale RL. Treinamento auditivo: avaliação da manutenção das habilidades. Pró-fono. 2002:14(1):93–8.

24 Gil D. Treinamento auditivo formal em adultos com deficiência auditiva. Dissertação apresentada à Universidade Federal de São Paulo para a obtenção do título de Mestre, São Paulo: Universidade Federal de São Paulo (UNIFESP). 2006.

9 Age-associated changes in cholesterol metabolism cardiovascular risk and exercise effect on lipid profile

Isabel Silva, Mariana Clemente, Carla Ferreira, Ana Margarida Silva, António Gabriel, Telmo Pereira, and Armando Caseiro

Introduction

Cholesterol is a steroid that plays several structural and metabolic roles that are vital to human biology and its metabolism, being affected with aging. The combination of cardiovascular risk factors like high serum cholesterol concentration and age call our attention. Appropriate prevention of chronic conditions and associated risk factors in old patients is critical to enable sustainable health care and maintain quality of life. Taking into account this major societal challenge, this chapter approaches several topics including cholesterol metabolism, the age-associated changes in cholesterol homeostasis and therapeutics, its relation with cardiovascular risk in this population as well as the effect of exercise on serum lipids.

Metabolism of cholesterol

Cholesterol is a long chain polycyclic alcohol, usually called a steroid, consisting of 27 carbons (C).[1] It plays several structural and metabolic roles vitals to human biology, being an important constituent of cell membranes in animals and crucial in their fluidity and permeability. It is also important to emphasize its importance as a precursor to steroid hormones and bile acids and is involved in transmembrane signaling and cell proliferation processes.[2]

In cell membranes, cholesterol molecules are interspersed between phospholipids, allowing for adequate membrane permeability as well as modulation of their fluidity at various physiological temperatures.[1]

DOI: 10.4324/9781003215271-9

It plays a crucial role in the formation of specialized domains rich in sphingolipids, such as lipid rafts and caveolae.[2] It also regulates the function of various membrane proteins through specific cholesterol–protein interactions and is also an important precursor in the biosynthesis of steroid hormones, oxysterols, and bile acids, responsible for specific and significant biological functions.[1,3]

Cholesterol is transported in plasma and the lipid profile describes the variable levels of lipids such as low-density lipoprotein (LDL) cholesterol, high density lipoprotein (HDL) cholesterol, total cholesterol (TC), and triglycerides (TG).[4] LDL is a lipoprotein responsible for transporting cholesterol to peripheral tissues, so increased levels of this marker are related to increased lipid deposition in vessels.[5–7] HDL is a lipoprotein capable of transporting cholesterol from peripheral areas to the liver for future use and elimination, thus having a protective function against cardiovascular disease (CVD) and prevention of atherosclerosis.[4,6] High serum TG levels are associated with a higher percentage of plasma lipids, so exacerbated levels of this marker are related to a higher percentage of visceral adipose tissue and consequent insulin resistance and other comorbidities.[8–10] Obesity, CVD, diabetes mellitus (DM) type 2 and atherosclerosis are characterized by high concentrations of LDL cholesterol, TC, TG, and low HDL cholesterol.[8,10,11]

Cholesterol absorption, synthesis and excretion contribute to the maintenance of cholesterol metabolism homeostasis. Exogenous cholesterol is absorbed in the intestine, while endogenous cholesterol is produced in both the liver and peripheral tissues. Cholesterol homeostasis is a process in which cholesterol levels are regulated in a controlled way by various endogenous and exogenous factors. To ensure maintenance of homeostasis, the body must integrate *de novo* cholesterol synthesis, uptake of circulating cholesterol (receptor-mediated), incorporation into cell membranes and lipoprotein secretion, as well as intracellular accumulation of cholesterol esters and the metabolism of oxysterols, bile salts, and steroid hormones.[1]

Cholesterol homeostasis is maintained by a feedback regulatory system that detects cholesterol levels in cell membranes and controls the transcription of genes encoding proteins involved in cholesterol synthesis and in post-transcription cholesterol-related events.[12]

An end product feedback repression occurs when cholesterol accumulates in cells, leading to LDL receptors (LDLr) gene repression in coordination with other genes encoding cholesterol biosynthesis enzymes.[13–15]

Cholesterol biosynthesis is regulated through a feedback inhibition system where intracellular cholesterol levels are detected, resulting in the modulation of expression of two membrane-incorporated endoplasmic reticulum (ER) proteins: sterol regulatory element binding protein 2 (SREBP-2) cleavage-activating protein (SCAP), and 3-hydroxy-3-methylglutaryl coenzyme-A (HMG-CoA) reductase.[16] These two proteins share an intramembrane sequence designed Sterol Sensing Domain (SSD). This domain is found in several proteins involved in cholesterol homeostasis.[2] In the presence of low cholesterol levels, the SREBP-2 forms a SREBP-2-SCAP complex, which binds to coat protein complex II (COP II). When cholesterol levels are then decreased in the ER membrane, this complex migrates through vesicles to the Golgi Complex apparatus. There SREBP-2 is cleaved by two proteases, S1P and S2P, the active domains being proteolytically released to enter the nucleus and activate the transcription of the genes encoding HMG-CoA reductase.[17–19] In the case of excess cholesterol, the SREBP-2-SCAP complex binds to an ER protein called insulin-induced gene 1 (INSIG-1). This binding prevents binding of COP II proteins. As a result, the SREBP-2-SCAP complex remains in the ER, the target gene transition decreases, with consequent decrease in cholesterol levels.[18]

In addition to SREBP, excess cholesterol is also detected by another transcription factor called liver X receptor (LXR), which is activated by sterol ligands such as oxysterols and certain intermediates in cholesterol synthesis.[20]

Body cholesterol is derived from two sources, *de novo* biosynthesis and diet. *De novo* synthesis is a complex metabolic cholesterol synthesis pathway from acetyl-CoA precursor unit. Generally, this pathway can be divided into two phases: (1) squalene phase, where squalene formation occurs through isoprenoid condensation; and (2) post-squalene phase, where squalene cyclization occurs to produce lanosterol, which is later converted to cholesterol.[16]

In the first phase, squalene phase, the two acetyl-CoA (2C) units are condensed due to the action of the thiolase enzyme, forming a acetoacetyl-CoA (4C) unit, to which a third acetyl-CoA unit is joined, leading to the formation of HMG-CoA (6C) by the action of the enzyme HMG-CoA synthase. HMG-CoA is converted to mevalonate (6C) by the action of the enzyme HMG-CoA reductase, an ER membrane glycoprotein considered a key enzyme in regulating cholesterol biosynthesis. The next step is characterized by the formation of the structural bases of the steroid cholesterol skeleton, the isoprenoids, which the base is the isopentenyl pyrophosphate (isopentenyl-PP) (5C) formed from mevalonate, by loss of carbon dioxide (CO_2). From isopentenyl-PP, geranyl pyrophosphate (geranyl-PP)

(10C) and farnesyl pyrophosphate (farnesyl-PP) (15C) are formed. The combination of two farnesyl-PP subunits results in squalene (30C) formation.[3]

Then, in a second phase, post-squalene phase of the cholesterol biosynthesis pathway, squalene is converted to lanosterol (30C), which will give rise to cholesterol (27C), through the action of various intermediate compounds, such as the case of zymosterol (27C), desmosterol (27C), and lathosterol (27C).[3]

With regard to cholesterol absorption, the process begins with the digestion and emulsification of dietary fats in the stomach by enzymatic action. Cholesterol enters the lumen of the small intestine through three sources: diet, bile and intestinal epithelial sloughing. The average daily intake of cholesterol in the western diet is approximately 300–500 mg and bile provides 800 to 1,200 mg of cholesterol per day. In turn, transformation of the intestinal mucosal epithelium establishes a third source of intraluminal cholesterol, which contributes about 300 mg of cholesterol per day. The main absorption sites are the duodenum and proximal jejunum.[21]

In healthy individuals, approximately 50% of intestinal cholesterol is absorbed.[22] Dietary cholesterol is partially esterified (<15%) compared to biliary cholesterol, which is predominantly unesterified. In these cases, dietary cholesteryl esters need to be de-esterified by the pancreatic carboxylic ester lipase enzyme before cholesterol is transported to the enterocytes.[3]

There are two enzymes mainly control the process of sterol uptake and intestinal transport: acetyl-CoA acetyltransferase (ACAT2) which facilitates intracellular esterification of cholesterol; and the microsomal triglyceride transfer protein (MTTP) which is involved in intestinal incorporation of chylomicrons.[23]

Among the proteins indicated as intestinal cholesterol carriers, it has recently been shown that Niemann-Pick C1Like 1 protein (NPC1L1) plays a critical role, expressed predominantly in the gastrointestinal tract, with maximum expression in the proximal jejunum.[2]

Export of cholesterol from enterocyte to the intestinal lumen requires expression of ATP-binding cassette (ABC) transporters. The ABC transporters, and in particular ABCG5 and ABCG8 act as functional heterodimers[24], and are located on the hepatocyte canalicular membrane and the enterocyte membrane. These transporters are the major components of the cholesterol reverse pathway and are critical for the efflux of cellular cholesterol excess. ABCG5 and ABCG8, in particular, represent the apical sterol cholesterol efflux of the enterocytes back into the intestinal lumen.[24]

After absorption by the enterocytes, cholesterol is accumulated as triglycerides in chylomicrons and subsequently secreted in lymph. In circulation, triglycerides are rapidly hydrolyzed and free fatty acids are absorbed into peripheral tissues. Cholesterol-enriched chylomicrons are later eliminated by the liver.[25]

Age-associated changes in cholesterol homeostasis

Aging is a physiological process characteristic of living beings influenced by the interaction of multiple endogenous and exogenous factors that characterize the adaptive biological response, and the genetic component.[26] This is characterized by loss of homeostasis that leads to changes in the biochemical composition of tissues, reduced adaptive responsiveness to environmental stimuli, and increased susceptibility and vulnerability to disease.[12,27] During the aging process, various aspects of cholesterol metabolism, including its synthesis and excretion, are compromised.[28]

Cholesterol homeostasis is maintained by LDLr mediated LDL endocytosis and *de novo* cholesterol synthesis through the enzyme HMG-CoA reductase as it is the limiting enzyme for conversion of HMG-CoA in mevalonate. This enzyme is targeted for cholesterol-lowering therapies like statins.[3,12,29] This regulation that ensures cholesterol homeostasis is fundamental and particularly strict, since cholesterol is essential in many cellular functions, however it can be toxic to the cell if present in excess.[30]

Several studies indicate that serum cholesterol levels increase in adulthood but tend to decrease in the older adult, thus it is important to know the effects of aging and the changes involved in the synthesis and consequently in cholesterol homeostasis.[31-33]

Choi et al.[28] conducted a study in rats and found a decrease in the activity of HMG-CoA reductase and cholesterol 7α-hydroxylase (C7α-OH) in adult rats compared to younger rats, related to a decrease in *de novo* cholesterol synthesis rate due to impairment of the enzyme that catalyzes the conversion of HMG-CoA to mevalonate as well as a decrease in cholesterol catabolism.

Human data are largely derived from the analysis of plasma levels of hydroxylated sterols, which are currently considered reliable markers of cholesterol absorption efficiency, such as sitosterol, lanosterol, and campesterol. A study by Bertolotti et al.[31] obtained similar results to the previous one where there was a reduction in cholesterol synthesis with aging. The finding may be related to a reduction in the metabolic requirement of cholesterol in old age, leading to a negative regulation of the main mechanisms of cholesterol intake in the liver. A trend of increase in plasma cholesterol with aging was observed in epidemiological studies, namely LDL cholesterol, however in very old age, a decrease in TC, and low cholesterol were observed, associated with poor health and multi-morbidity.[31,34,35]

Other studies have been performed with results contradicting the previous findings. The study by Stahlberg et al.[36] reported a marked decrease in hepatic HMG-CoA reductase activity in rats between 1 and 6 months of age, however the activity remained essentially unchanged during adulthood. C7α-OH activity decreased gradually with age, as found in studies by Choi et al. and Bertolotti et al., suggesting that the decline in activity of this enzyme, which reflects a decrease in the ability to metabolize cholesterol to bile acids, may contribute to increased plasma cholesterol in old age. HMG-CoA reductase activity, which remains relatively stable despite increased liver cholesterol levels, may indicate that regulation of synthesis becomes slower with age.[36]

Further evidence demonstrates that in addition to the decreased ability of cholesterol conversion to bile acids as a result of the decline of the C7α-OH, the causes of age-related lipid homeostasis rupture include the gradual decline of fractional clearance of LDL. In addition, a hypothesis states that critical changes in cholesterol and lipoprotein metabolism depend on the progressive decrease in growth hormone secretion. This hormone plays an important role in cholesterol homeostasis by modulating hepatic LDLr expression and controlling C7α-OH activity.[12]

Cholesterol and cardiovascular risk in older patients

Appropriate prevention of chronic conditions such as CVD and associated risk factors in older patients is becoming increasingly important to enable sustainable health care and maintain quality of life, especially in the older population. Age represents an important determinant of cardiovascular risk and is perhaps the most relevant determinant when considering coronary heart disease. Other risk factors for which treatment options are available include systolic blood pressure, circulating cholesterol levels, smoking and DM.[37]

When considering the effects of aging and cholesterol on cardiovascular risk, together with the wide availability of safe and effective pharmacological cholesterol lowering agents, it is assumed that this treatment is highly recommended for the older population. However, in this population there are other aspects to consider, such as age-related changes in pharmacokinetic and pharmacodynamic properties of drugs, predisposing to drug-associated adverse events and/or pharmacological interactions.[37,38]

The main goal of cholesterol-lowering treatments is to provide significant protection for these individuals; however, direct experimental evidence is very limited, especially in the older strata of the population.[37] Age-related changes in cholesterol metabolism are still poorly defined, in part due to the scarcity of direct experimental data on lipid pathophysiology.[39]

Age and plasma cholesterol concentration are well-recognized cardiovascular risk factors, according to different functions designed to provide a quantitative estimate of the possibility of total or fatal cardiovascular events.[40–43]

Studies report a lower relative impact of cholesterol in older age groups, where age itself tends to prevail over other risk factors.[44,45] In some studies, low TC and LDL cholesterol have even been found to be associated with worse cardiovascular outcomes and all-cause mortality.[46] This phenomenon, called reverse epidemiology, is explained by the possibility that low levels of a given risk factor are not a cause, but a consequence of underlying conditions – such as chronic disease or cancer – that compromise general health status, leading to worse results.[47] In particular, low levels of HDL cholesterol were considered to be a recognized risk factor for cognitive impairment in the older population.[48]

The impact of different variables may not be constant across all age groups and the coefficients for the individual risk factors used in these algorithms may not be adequate in that scenario. Indeed, well-established risk functions for younger people appear to perform worse in old and very old adults.[49] To overcome these limitations, a new risk estimation function was calculated and validated for the older age groups in the European Systematic Coronary Risk Assessment (SCORE) dataset, called SCORE OP, to quantify the individual risk of a fatal cardiovascular event. This function includes widely recognized risk factors such as gender, smoking, DM as dichotomous variables and age, TC and systolic blood pressure as numerical variables.[40,50]

This approach has important clinical implications because a more accurate definition of individual risk may prevent overtreatment and reduce unnecessary drug exposure in older patients given the high risk of drug-related events and interactions. The quantitative estimate of risk over 80 years of age remains an unresolved issue.[37]

Overall, at this time, there do not seem to be exhaustive guidelines implemented for the control of hypercholesterolemia in the older population. Therefore, the administration of a pharmacological treatment and the proper selection of the indicated drug should be tailored to each patient and aspects should be considered such as patient frailty, disability, and age.[37]

Effect of exercise on serum lipids

The health of the population is an important factor in the quality of life of individuals.[51] Obesity is an epidemiological disease that affects the health of any age range[52,53] due to heterogeneous etiology such as: high fat diet, genetic susceptibility, sedentary lifestyle among other factors. Obesity is associated with DM type 2, high blood pressure, dyslipidemia, atherosclerosis, all causes that increase the risk of CVD.[54-56]

CVD are the leading causes of death worldwide. Physical inactivity is considered one of the risk factors that contribute to increased incidence and prevalence.[57] Prevention of these pathologies and comorbidities involves not only the acquisition of a healthy diet and weight, but also physical exercise, which can be verified through some studies that report beneficial effects on the lipid profile.[4,58,59]

In recent years, several studies have increasingly described the importance of physical exercise in health, in prevention of comorbidities and in of decrease mortality. Exercise can be practiced regardless of age, gender and can be practiced as sport or leisure. Data from several studies describe the benefits of regular physical exercise in cognitive and mental health by promoting loss of body fat mass, increasing lean body mass, cognitive function, decreasing cases of DM type 2, gestational diabetes, hypertension, improvement of emotional disorders, mood, protective action against dementia, among others.[60-63]

Several studies suggest changes in lipid profile depending on the type, amount and intensity of physical exercise performed regardless of diet. One of the notable lipid differences between sedentary and active individuals is the c-HDL level.[62,64] On average about 25–30% of the energy used daily is consumed by muscle activity. Muscle activity is the way which more energy is consumed leading to a reduction in TG reserves. Thus, during exercise there is greater mobilization and metabolization of lipids as opposed to glycogen at the muscle level, thereby reducing plasma lipid levels.[6]

Such mechanisms may be explained by some studies describing increased lecithin cholesterol acyltransferase (LCAT), reduced cholesterol ester transfer protein (CETP) and or increased lipoprotein lipase (LPL) activity. The enzyme LCAT is responsible for esterification of plasma cholesterol. In fact, one study has shown increased levels of LCAT after exercise. The increase of this enzyme leads to a decrease in cholesterol levels in peripheral tissues by increasing HDL cholesterol particles.[6,65] Some authors have analyzed the effect of exercise intensity and frequency and while some authors observed that HDL cholesterol increases regardless of intensity and frequency, others found that only the high intensity and high frequency group had a significant increase in HDL cholesterol concentration.[59,65-67]

The CETP enzyme is responsible for the transfer of HDL cholesterol to other lipoproteins. Its reduction leads to lower cholesterol in peripheral tissues.[64,67,68] The LPL is a group of enzymes, that belong to a family of hydrolytic enzymes that play a key role in increasing HDL cholesterol levels due to exercise.[64] In contrast, some studies have not shown changes in HDL cholesterol levels, reporting only variations when there are changes in body mass.[59,69] Other studies have shown that regular exercise leads to a decrease in HDL cholesterol levels regardless of the intensity, frequency or type of exercise, however it is necessary to exclude potential interference such as weight loss, dietary changes, and others.[58]

In a study, a group of individuals with nonalcoholic hepatic steatosis, when undergoing physical exercise lasting 12 weeks without weight loss, showed results of reduced hepatic fat, visceral fat and TG levels and there was an increase in % MM.[70] A study on the practice of physical exercise during pregnancy has shown overall maternal and neonatal benefits, reducing the risk of hypertension, gestational diabetes, excess weight and improvements in maternal lipid profile with reduction of LDL cholesterol, CT and TG levels and higher HDL cholesterol levels.[71,72] A sedentary behavior, also in pregnant women, showed worse results.[73] According to Prado et al.[69] no significant changes in lipid profile were found in the practice of strength exercises.

As mentioned before, uncontrolled high levels of LDL cholesterol have detrimental effects on the health of individuals. It is essential to devise strategies for its reduction.[64] One way to reduce LDL cholesterol is through drug therapy such as statins.[6] The authors concluded that the risk of mortality is significantly lower when statin therapy is combined with exercise compared to either method alone.[64]

Exercise leads to increased LPL activity in the muscles. In fact, exercise depletes the TG content, thereby inducing LPL synthesis, with subsequent TG hydrolysis by LPL and transfer of cholesterol to HDL, which leads to further catabolism of TG-rich lipoproteins, thereby forming fewer LDL particles. Still, reducing CETP appears to reduce LDL formation, so there is less lipid deposition in peripheral tissues.[64,67,68] However, the effect of exercise on lipids and lipoproteins is not yet fully understood and further studies are needed to reduce interference such as weight loss, dietary changes and others in order to study the changes in lipid profile.[10]

Conclusion

Serum cholesterol levels change over the lifetime, increasing in adulthood but tending to decrease in the older adult, being important to know the effects of aging in cholesterol homeostasis. Age and blood cholesterol concentration are well-recognized cardiovascular risk factors, although no exhaustive guidelines for the control of hypercholesterolemia in the older population are available. In fact, regular exercise improves lipid profile and the quality of life of individuals, regardless of age. The practice of physical exercise combined with other therapies such as diet and drugs lead to more significant changes in lipid profile. Therefore, the administration of a pharmacological treatment and the proper selection of the drug should be tailored to each patient. Also physical exercise should be prescribed in a personalized way, particularly in the older adult. Considering the effects of cholesterol and aging on cardiovascular risk and the availability of safe and effective lipid lowering agents the treatment is highly recommended for the older population.

Key points

- Serum cholesterol levels change with aging.
- Age and blood cholesterol concentration are well-recognized cardiovascular risk factors.
- Uncontrolled high levels of LDL cholesterol have detrimental effects on the health of individuals.
- Regular physical exercise improves lipid profile.
- The treatment with cholesterol lowering agents is highly recommendable for older adults.

References

1 Rezen, T., et al., Interplay between cholesterol and drug metabolism. Biochim Biophys Acta, 2011. 1814(1): p. 146–60.
2 Martini, C. and V. Pallottini, Cholesterol: from feeding to gene regulation. Genes Nutr, 2007. 2(2): p. 181–93.

3　van der Wulp, M.Y., H.J. Verkade, and A.K. Groen, Regulation of cholesterol homeostasis. Mol Cell Endocrinol, 2013. 368(1–2): p. 1–16.

4　Mann, S., C. Beedie, and A. Jimenez, Differential effects of aerobic exercise, resistance training and combined exercise modalities on cholesterol and the lipid profile: review, synthesis and recommendations. Sports Med, 2014. 44(2): p. 211–21.

5　Tian, J., et al., Trends in the levels of serum lipids and lipoproteins and the prevalence of dyslipidemia in adults with newly diagnosed type 2 diabetes in the Southwest Chinese Han population during 2003–2012. Int J Endocrinol, 2015. 2015: p. 818075.

6　Guyton, A.C. and A.C.G. John E. Hall, Tratado de fisiologia Medica. Amsterdam: Elsevier, 2006.

7　Whelton, S.P., et al., Relation of isolated low high-density lipoprotein cholesterol to mortality and cardiorespiratory fitness (from the Henry Ford Exercise Testing Project [FIT project]). Am J Cardiol, 2019. 123(9): p. 1429–34.

8　Malik, S.U.F., et al., Relationship among obesity, blood lipids and insulin resistance in Bangladeshi adults. Diabetes Metab Syndr, 2019. 13(1): p. 444–9.

9　Hernandez-Lepe, M.A., et al., Double-blind randomised controlled trial of the independent and synergistic effect of Spirulina maxima with exercise (ISESE) on general fitness, lipid profile and redox status in overweight and obese subjects: study protocol. BMJ Open, 2017. 7(6): p. e013744.

10　Branco, B.H.M., et al., Effects of the order of physical exercises on body composition, physical fitness, and cardiometabolic risk in adolescents participating in an interdisciplinary program focusing on the treatment of obesity. Front Physiol, 2019. 10: p. 1013.

11　Baran, J., et al., Blood lipid profile and body composition in a pediatric population with different levels of physical activity. Lipids Health Dis, 2018. 17(1): p. 171.

12　Trapani, L. and V. Pallottini, Age-related hypercholesterolemia and HMG-CoA reductase dysregulation: sex does matter (a gender perspective). Curr Gerontol Geriatrics Res, 2010. 2010: p. 420139.

13　Brown, M.S. and J.L. Goldstein, Regulation of the activity of the low density lipoprotein receptor in human fibroblasts. Cell, 1975. 6(3): p. 307–16.

14　Brown, M.S. and J.L. Goldstein, Cholesterol feedback: from Schoenheimer's bottle to Scap's MELADL. J Lipid Res, 2009. 50 Suppl: p. S15–27.

15　Brown, M.S., A. Radhakrishnan, and J.L. Goldstein, Retrospective on cholesterol homeostasis: the central role of SCAP. Annu Rev Biochem, 2018. 87: p. 783–807.

16　Alphonse, P.A. and P.J. Jones, Revisiting human cholesterol synthesis and absorption: the reciprocity paradigm and its key regulators. Lipids, 2016. 51(5): p. 519–36.

17 Matsuda, M., et al., SREBP cleavage-activating protein (SCAP) is required for increased lipid synthesis in liver induced by cholesterol deprivation and insulin elevation. Genes Dev, 2001. 15(10): p. 1206–16.

18 Radhakrishnan, A., et al., Switch-like control of SREBP-2 transport triggered by small changes in ER cholesterol: a delicate balance. Cell Metab, 2008. 8(6): p. 512–21.

19 Goldstein, J.L., R.A. DeBose-Boyd, and M.S. Brown, Protein sensors for membrane sterols. Cell, 2006. 124(1): p. 35–46.

20 Gelissen, I.C. and A.J. Brown, An overview of cholesterol homeostasis. Methods Mol Biol, 2017. 1583: p. 1–6.

21 Lammert, F. and D.Q. Wang, New insights into the genetic regulation of intestinal cholesterol absorption. Gastroenterology, 2005. 129(2): p. 718–34.

22 Sudhop, T., et al., Inhibition of intestinal cholesterol absorption by ezetimibe in humans. Circulation, 2002. 106(15): p. 1943–8.

23 Wang, D.Q., Regulation of intestinal cholesterol absorption. Annu Rev Physiol, 2007. 69: p. 221–48.

24 Graf, G.A., et al., Coexpression of ATP-binding cassette proteins ABCG5 and ABCG8 permits their transport to the apical surface. J Clin Invest, 2002. 110(5): p. 659–69.

25 Kruit, J.K., et al., Emerging roles of the intestine in control of cholesterol metabolism. World J Gastroenterol, 2006. 12(40): p. 6429–39.

26 Bron, D., et al., Aging and blood disorders: new perspectives, new challenges. Haematologica, 2015. 100(4): p. 415–7.

27 Marino, M., et al., Age-related changes of cholesterol and dolichol biosynthesis in rat liver. Mech Ageing Dev, 2002. 123(8): p. 1183–9.

28 Choi, Y.S., T. Ide, and M. Sugano, Age-related changes in the regulation of cholesterol metabolism in rats. Exp Gerontol, 1987. 22(5): p. 339–49.

29 Goedeke, L. and C. Fernandez-Hernando, Regulation of cholesterol homeostasis. Cell Mol Life Sci, 2012. 69(6): p. 915–30.

30 Mulas, M.F., et al., Dietary restriction counteracts age-related changes in cholesterol metabolism in the rat. Mech Ageing Dev, 2005. 126(6–7): p. 648–54.

31 Bertolotti, M., et al., Age-associated alterations in cholesterol homeostasis: evidence from a cross-sectional study in a Northern Italy population. Clin Interv Aging, 2014. 9: p. 425–32.

32 Wilson, P.W., et al., Determinants of change in total cholesterol and HDL-C with age: the Framingham Study. J Gerontol, 1994. 49(6): p. M252–7.

33 Cohen, J.D., et al., 30-year trends in serum lipids among United States adults: results from the National Health and Nutrition Examination Surveys II, III, and 1999–2006. Am J Cardiol, 2010. 106(7): p. 969–75.

34 Galman, C., B. Angelin, and M. Rudling, Pronounced variation in bile acid synthesis in humans is related to gender, hypertriglyceridaemia and circulating levels of fibroblast growth factor 19. J Intern Med, 2011. 270(6): p. 580–8.

35 Tilvis, R.S., et al., Prognostic significance of serum cholesterol, lathosterol, and sitosterol in old age; a 17-year population study. Ann Med, 2011. 43(4): p. 292–301.

36 Stahlberg, D., B. Angelin, and K. Einarsson, Age-related changes in the metabolism of cholesterol in rat liver microsomes. Lipids, 1991. 26(5): p. 349–52.

37 Bertolotti, M., G. Lancellotti, and C. Mussi, Management of high cholesterol levels in older people. Geriatr Gerontol Int, 2019. 19(5): p. 375–83.

38 Szadkowska, I., et al., Statin therapy in the elderly: a review. Arch Gerontol Geriatr, 2010. 50(1): p. 114–8.

39 Morgan, A.E., et al., Cholesterol metabolism: a review of how ageing disrupts the biological mechanisms responsible for its regulation. Ageing Res Rev, 2016. 27: p. 108–24.

40 Conroy, R.M., et al., Estimation of ten-year risk of fatal cardiovascular disease in Europe: the SCORE project. Eur Heart J, 2003. 24(11): p. 987–1003.

41 Giampaoli, S., et al., The global cardiovascular risk chart. Ital Heart J Suppl, 2004. 5(3): p. 177–85.

42 Assmann, G., P. Cullen, and H. Schulte, Simple scoring scheme for calculating the risk of acute coronary events based on the 10-year follow-up of the prospective cardiovascular Munster (PROCAM) study. Circulation, 2002. 105(3): p. 310–5.

43 Goff, D.C., Jr., et al., 2013 ACC/AHA guideline on the assessment of cardiovascular risk: a report of the American College of Cardiology/American Heart Association Task Force on Practice Guidelines. J Am Coll Cardiol, 2014. 63(25 Pt B): p. 2935–59.

44 Prospective Studies, C., et al., Blood cholesterol and vascular mortality by age, sex, and blood pressure: a meta-analysis of individual data from 61 prospective studies with 55,000 vascular deaths. Lancet, 2007. 370(9602): p. 1829–39.

45 Catapano, A.L., et al., 2016 ESC/EAS guidelines for the management of dyslipidaemias. Eur Heart J, 2016. 37(39): p. 2999–3058.

46 Schupf, N., et al., Relationship between plasma lipids and all-cause mortality in nondemented elderly. J Am Geriatr Soc, 2005. 53(2): p. 219–26.

47 Ahmadi, S.F., et al., Reverse epidemiology of traditional cardiovascular risk factors in the geriatric population. J Am Med Dir Assoc, 2015. 16(11): p. 933–9.

48. Zuliani, G., et al., Relationship between low levels of high-density lipoprotein cholesterol and dementia in the elderly. The InChianti Study. J Gerontol A Biol Sci Med Sci, 2010. 65(5): p. 559–64.

49 Stork, S., et al., Prediction of mortality risk in the elderly. Am J Med, 2006. 119(6): p. 519–25.

50 Cooney, M.T., et al., Cardiovascular risk estimation in older persons: SCORE O.P. Eur J Prev Cardiol, 2016. 23(10): p. 1093–103.

51 Mehta, N. and M. Myrskyla, The population health benefits of a healthy lifestyle: life expectancy increased and onset of disability delayed. Health Aff (Millwood), 2017. 36:(8): p. 1495–502.

52 Costantino, S., et al. Epigenetic processing in cardiometabolic disease. Atherosclerosis, 2018. DOI: 10.1016/j.atherosclerosis.2018.09.029.

53 Chade, A.R. and J.E. Hall, Role of the renal microcirculation in progression of chronic kidney injury in obesity. Am J Nephrol, 2016. 44(5): p. 354–67.

54 Turner, P.A., et al., Spheroid culture system confers differentiated transcriptome profile and functional advantage to 3T3-L1 adipocytes. Ann Biomed Eng, 2018. 46(5): p. 772–87.

55 Sfyri, P.P., et al., Attenuation of oxidative stress-induced lesions in skeletal muscle in a mouse model of obesity-independent hyperlipidaemia and atherosclerosis through the inhibition of Nox2 activity. Free Radic Biol Med, 2018. 129: p. 504–19.

56 Mavilio, M., et al., A role for Timp3 in microbiota-driven hepatic steatosis and metabolic dysfunction. Cell Rep, 2016. 16(3): p. 731–43.

57 Lavie, C.J., et al., Sedentary behavior, exercise, and cardiovascular health. Circ Res, 2019. 124(5): p. 799–815.

58 Chooi, Y.C., et al., Lipoprotein subclass profile after progressive energy deficits induced by calorie restriction or exercise. Nutrients, 2018. 10(11): p. 1814.

59 Trejo-Gutierrez, J.F. and G. Fletcher, Impact of exercise on blood lipids and lipoproteins. J Clin Lipidol, 2007. 1(3): p. 175–81.

60 Rego, M.L., et al., Physical exercise for individuals with hypertension: it is time to emphasize its benefits on the brain and cognition. Clin Med Insights Cardiol, 2019. 13: p. 1179546819839411.

61 Achi, N.K., et al., Modulation of the lipid profile and insulin levels of streptozotocin induced diabetic rats by ethanol extract of *Cnidoscolus aconitifolius* leaves and some fractions: Effect on the oral glucose tolerance of normoglycemic rats. Biomed Pharmacother, 2017. 86: p. 562–69.

62 Takehara, K., et al., The effectiveness of exercise intervention for academic achievement, cognitive function, and physical health among children in Mongolia: a cluster RCT study protocol. BMC Public Health, 2019. 19(1): p. 697.

63 Chan, J.S.Y., et al., Special Issue – Therapeutic benefits of physical activity for mood: a systematic review on the effects of exercise intensity, duration, and modality. J Psychol, 2019. 153(1): p. 102–25.

64 Wang, Y. and D. Xu, Effects of aerobic exercise on lipids and lipoproteins. Lipids Health Dis, 2017. 16(1): p. 132.

65 Cox, R.A. and M.R. Garcia-Palmieri, Cholesterol, triglycerides, and associated lipoproteins, in: Walker, H.K., W.D. Hall, J.W. Hurst (Eds.), Clinical Methods: The History, Physical, and Laboratory Examinations, 3rd ed. Boston, MA: Butterworths. 1990.

66 Igarashi, Y. and Y. Nogami, Response of lipids and lipoproteins to regular aquatic endurance exercise: a meta-analysis of randomized controlled trials. J Atheroscler Thromb, 2019. 26(1): p. 14–30.

67 Leança, C.C., et al., HDL: o yin-yang da doença cardiovascular. Arquivos Brasileiros de Endocrinologia & Metabologia, 2010. 54: p. 777–84.

68 Lee, M., et al., Studies on the plasma lipid profiles, and LCAT and CETP activities according to hyperlipoproteinemia phenotypes (HLP). Atherosclerosis, 2001. 159(2): p. 381–9.

69 Prado, E.S. and E.H.M. Dantas, Efeitos dos exercícios físicos aeróbio e de força nas lipoproteínas HDL, LDL e lipoproteína(a). Arq Bras Cardiol, 2002. 79: p. 429–33.

70 Houghton, D., et al., Exercise reduces liver lipids and visceral adiposity in patients with nonalcoholic steatohepatitis in a randomized controlled trial. Clin Gastroenterol Hepatol, 2017. 15(1): p. 96–102.e3.

71 Ramirez-Velez, R., et al., Exercise during pregnancy on maternal lipids: a secondary analysis of randomized controlled trial. BMC Pregnancy Childb, 2017. 17(1): p. 396.

72 Bo, S., et al., Simple lifestyle recommendations and the outcomes of gestational diabetes. A 2 x 2 factorial randomized trial. Diabetes Obes Metab, 2014. 16(10): p. 1032–5.

73 Szumilewicz, A., et al., Acute postexercise change in circulating irisin is related to more favorable lipid profile in pregnant women attending a structured exercise program and to less favorable lipid profile in controls: an experimental study with two groups. Int J Endocrinol, 2019. 2019: p. 1932503.

10 Impact of a multidisciplinary intervention program on skeletal muscle in the older adult

Rute Santos

Introduction

Worldwide, the population is getting older and older. This phenomenon presents challenges and opportunities. On the one hand, it leads to an increase in basic health care and long-term care, appropriate environments, while on the other, it brings a closer look at the global health-related entities, revealing concern about the need to implement strategies to promote health care, active aging and a better quality of life through community intervention programs. The use of evaluation methods provides evidence of the benefits of these programs in attenuating musculoskeletal disorders caused by aging. Thus, allowing society to invest in healthy aging provides individuals with a longer, autonomous, and healthy life.

Demographic aging in Portugal

In recent decades, Portugal, like other countries in Europe, has presented an aging demographic structure. Associated with this growing aging population, there is a reduction in births and the young population[1,2]. In 2015, the population aged 65 and over represented 20.5% of the entire resident population in Portugal. That same year, life expectancy reached 77.4 years for men and 83.2 years for women[2]. According to the National Institute of Statistics (INE), in 2012, the aging pattern of the population is continuing, and the number of older people will reach its highest value by the end of 2040s, having a strong impact on society at various levels, including health, education, and others[3-5].

Aging process

The definition of the concept of aging has been changing due to a greater anatomophysiological knowledge and, on the other hand,

DOI: 10.4324/9781003215271-10

to the shift of social thoughts and behaviors[6]. However, it can be broadly defined as an active, continuous and differential process that encompasses physical, biological, psychological and social changes, that influence the social definition of the person throughout life[6-9]. Although chronological age is broadly accepted as the criterion for the definition of aging, aging is a much more complex and multidimensional concept, and therefore chronological age should not be considered alone to evaluate the human development[6,7,9]. According to the World Health Organization, the definition of the older adult begins between the ages of 60 and 65[6,10]. However, individuals of the same chronological age are not necessarily in the same aging stages, since it depends on biological, psychological, and social factors[6,10,11].

The aging process can then be considered singular and progressive, regarding the rhythm and form of manifestation, although natural and universal to all, and this heterogeneity can be explained by the interaction of genetic factors with environmental and cultural circumstances[6,12]. In this sense and according to several authors, the aging process results from three elements: biological, social, and psychological[6,7,13]. The biological element reflects an organic aging, where body structures change, causing greater vulnerability and disability of the individual. The social element represents the expectations of society for these individuals. The psychological element, on the other hand, is defined by the alteration of behavioral competences, encompassing the cognitive part of the individual, namely intelligence, memory, and motivation[6,13] (Table 10.1).

Table 10.1 Aging process: biological, psychological, and social dimensions

	Characteristics
Biological aging	• Progressive loss of functionality and adaptation or resistance to stress
	• Organism vulnerability and gradual likelihood of death
	• Adaptability to maintain homeostasis (depending on age)
Psychological aging	• Changes associated with the intellectual aspect and individual's life history
	• Adaptation of the individual's capacity for psychological self-regulation (in relation to the biological component)
Social aging	• Adaptation of the interaction pattern between the individual's life cycle and the social structure in which they are inserted
	• Behavioral performance of the individual and social expectations (depending on age)
	• Assignment of new norms, positions, opportunities, or restrictions to the individual (depending on age)

The effects of aging on the body

With aging, many changes occur in the human body regarding its morphology and physiology or functionality (Table 10.2). These changes can occur at various levels, specially the endocrine, digestive, urinary, immunological, nervous, anthropometric, respiratory, cardiovascular systems[13], reducing motor skills, flexibility, strength and speed, making it difficult to perform activities, and maintaining a healthy lifestyle[13,14].

Table 10.2 Structural changes resulting from aging and clinical manifestations

Organ or system	Structural changes with age	Clinical manifestations
Anthropometric level	Decreased height; Weight gain	Decreased arches of the feet; Increased curvature of the spine by alteration of intervertebral discs; Increased diameter of skull and rib cage; Decrease in fat free mass; Increased body fat; Decreased muscle mass; Decreased bone density.
Renal system	Decrease in the number of nephrons; Tubular dysfunction; Decreased bladder tone and capacity; Reduction of sphincter tone; Prostatic hyperplasia; Pelvic Muscle Hypotonia	Reduction of glomerular filtration rate; Decreased tubular absorption; Obstructive uropathy; Strain incontinence; Stress incontinence (mechanical).
Cardiovascular system	Reduction of cardiomyocytes; Decreased ventricular distensibility; Decreased elasticity of vessels; Increased vascular resistance; Baroreceptor Sensitivity Reduction	Decreased systolic volume; Decreased use of O_2 by tissues; Decreased heart rate; Decreased cardiac reserve; Increased pulse pressure; Arterial hypertension; Orthostatic hypotension; Repeating syncope; Less ability to adapt and recover from exercise; Increased O_2 Output

Muscle aging

As previously described, human aging is associated with a significant decline in neuromuscular function and performance. Sarcopenia is defined as an age-associated condition of muscle degeneration that is clearly related to decreased anabolic stimulation with aging, that is, a geriatric syndrome characterized by progressive decrease in muscle mass, strength and function[15,16]. Sarcopenia is caused by an imbalance between signs of muscle cell growth and signs of disintegration, and includes the effects of altered central and peripheral nervous system innervation, altered hormonal status, altered caloric and protein intake, and inflammatory effects[15–17]. All these factors contribute to sarcopenia and the characteristic atrophy and weakness of the skeletal muscle, which are considered the main contributing factors to the loss of functional mobility, independence and fragility present in many older people[16,18,19]. This condition can lead to negative impacts, especially in a higher risk of falls, hospitalizations, dependence, institutionalization, decreased quality of life and mortality, having a great social and economic impact[18].

It is known that from 20/30 years to 80 years there is a 30% reduction in muscle mass and 20% reduction in muscle cross-sectional area, being more noticeable in lower limb muscle groups, where the vastus lateralis transverse area may be reduced by up to 40%[17]. This decrease becomes more evident from the age of 50 where a decline in skeletal muscle mass of approximately 8% per decade to age 70 is observed and about 15% over the following decades. On the other hand, the decline in fat-free mass is twice as high in men compared to women and is amplified in sedentary individuals as compared to those who are physically active. In parallel, muscle strength decreases 10–15% per decade up to 70 years, later increasing to 25–40% every 10 years[19,17]. Associated with this decrease, changes occur in the quality of muscle fibers and also in architecture of the skeletal muscle, notably in the dimensions of the muscle fascicles and the angle of pennation[19–21].

Diagnosis of structural changes in the human body

There are several methods available for measuring muscle mass, including imaging methods such as computed tomography, magnetic resonance imaging, dual energy radiographic absorptiometry (DEXA) and ultrasound. Availability, cost and limitations differ among the various methods, with the DEXA technique being the method of choice, however unhelpful regarding its portability.

Ultrasonography, for its part, has shown, through several studies, to be an examination with great sensitivity and specificity to evaluate muscle morphology and architecture[22–24]. On the other hand, it has several advantages, namely its portability, cost and non-use of ionizing radiation[25].

Muscle ultrasound assessment

Regarding muscle ultrasound evaluation, there are several parameters that can be considered, the most commonly used: eco-intensity (EI), eco-structure, contour, and dimensions (i.e. thickness), in order to evaluate muscle morphological changes and tendons, caused by pathologies or physiological aspects. As such, thickness and EI are increasingly analyzed parameters associated with muscle function and muscle mechanics[26].

Muscle thickness (MT) is defined as the distance between the most superficial aponeurosis and the deepest muscle aponeurosis, obtained from B-mode muscle ultrasound images and is highly correlated with the muscle cross-sectional area[27–30]. It is a quantitative parameter that can be obtained in transverse and longitudinal planes to evaluate chronic muscle adaptations to different strength training protocols, being associated with muscle strength[30,31]. Muraki defends MT as an accurate and predictive parameter of muscle strength, however there is still some controversy regarding the cross-sectional area of muscles[32]. EI, in turn, is defined by the average intensity of pixels within the muscle of interest, usually using a gray level scale within a given region of interest. Although some studies confirm the good inter-session reliability of muscle EI measurements, some questions remain, namely about the size of the region of interest[33,34]. Santos et al. showed that ultrasound measurements of MT and muscle IE have moderate to very high reliability, its reliability and agreement being improved in the transverse plane and with larger regions of interest[30].

Musculoskeletal ultrasound and aging

Diagnostic imaging methods allow the diagnosis and follow-up of pathological, morphological and physiological changes, particularly allowing the assessment and monitoring of aging and muscle development[8]. Musculoskeletal ultrasound enables the identification of muscle morphological changes caused by effects of aging and/or physical activity[35].

Active aging

As a consequence of population aging, the World Health Organization has shown great concern about the need to implement "Active Aging" policies and programs, specially, physical activity, in order to reduce the effects of aging, always based on rights, needs, preferences and skills of the older adult, in order to provide the older population with a more active, healthy and participative life, thus providing a better quality of life for these individuals and their families[7].

According to the literature, physical activity in the older population has physical, functional, and physiological benefits and helps in the prevention of diseases resulting from the aging process[8]. In the light of this concern and the World Health Organization recommendations, the responsible entities have been promoting changes in behaviors and attitudes, proper training of health professionals and other professionals involved in social intervention, and the adaptation of health and social support services to the new social and family circumstances that convoy with aging[12,36].

Intervention programs and their benefits

Physical activity

Acknowledging the effects of population aging, particularly on the individual functionality, mobility and health, leading to decreased autonomy in their daily activities and consequently decreasing their quality of life,[9,37] it is essential to sensitize the population to the long-term benefits of an active life and the regular practice of physical activity. Several studies strongly support the association of healthy eating and regular physical activity with the attenuation of the degenerative changes within aging, encompassing the physical, psychological and social domains[9,37,38].

The AGA@4life approach

The AGA@4life project, similarly to other intervention programs, aims to encourage a thorough evaluation, monitorization and intervention in the older adult, implementing strategies that promote healthier lifestyle but respecting the individual specificities, needs and motivations. This project's original approach relies on the integration of a holistic and multidisciplinary assessment, aimed at mapping the health status of the older adult, considering the individual needs identified in a comprehensive diagnostic assessment and the expectations of the person. This intervention model promotes physical activity and functionality, fall prevention, nutritional optimization, cognitive stimulation, auditory training and promotion of psychosocial well-being. With regard to the preliminary results of the muscle ultrasound assessment, it was verified, in line with previous research, that an improvement of the muscle morphology of the old adult submitted to a tailored physical activity program and nutritional adjustment[7,35,37,39–41]. Changes in MT and eco-intensity were observed, showing attenuation of musculoskeletal changes caused by aging, namely in increasing MT and decreased eco-intensity, anticipating promising results in improving some aspects of functional autonomy overall throughout life.

Conclusions

As society is increasingly aging and considering the musculoskeletal changes inherent to this process, the preliminary results of the AGA@4life approach corroborate the need for a comprehensive assessment of the old adult's health and the implementation of strategies and the design and implementation of tailored intervention programs in order to reduce the aging impact on the population's quality of life. Consequently, projects like this should be available in dedicated institutions, such as day centers and nursing homes, amongst others, in order to make older people and health professionals aware of active and healthy aging in a multidisciplinary approach.

Key points

- Aging is an active and continuous process that causes morphological and physiological changes over the musculoskeletal system.
- Physical activity associated with healthy eating promotes attenuation of the musculoskeletal changes caused by aging.

References

1   Caipiro A. Envelhecimento e Dinâmicas Sociais. (Trabalho de Licenciatura). 2012.

2   PORDATA. Retrato de Portugal Na Europa. Edição 201. 2015.

3   INE. Estatísticas Demográficas 2012. 2013th ed. (Instituito Nacional de Estatística I, ed.). 2013.

4 INE. Projeções de População Residente 2015–2080. Inst Nac Estatística. 2017.

5 Moreira M. O envelhecimento da população e o seu impacto na habitação – Prospectiva Até 2050. (Tese de Mestrado). 2008.

6 Azevedo M. O envelhecimento ativo e a qualidade de vida: uma revisão integrativa. 2015.

7 Santos R. Programa de Intervenção em idosos: atividade física, autonomia funcional e qualidade de vida Programa de Intervenção em idosos: atividade física, autonomia funcional e qualidade de vida. 2014.

8 Fechine B, Trompieri N. O Processo de Envelhecimento: as principais alterações que acontecem com o idoso com o passar dos anos. Rev Científica Int. 2012;1(1):106–132.

9 Rocha S. Efeitos do aumento da atividade física na funcionalidade e qualidade das pessoas idosas do Centro Social de Ermesinde. (Relatório de Estágio de Mestrado). 2012.

10 Cancela M. O processo de envelhecimento 2007. (Relatório de estágio de Licenciatura). psicologia.com.pt. Published 2008.

11 Matsudo S, Keihan V, Matsudo R, Neto T. Impacto do envelhecimento nas variáveis antropométricas, neuromotoras e metabólicas da aptidão física. Rev Bras Ciência e Mov. 2000;8(4):21–32.

12 Cerqueira M. Imagens do envelhecimento e da velhice – Um estudo na população portuguesa. (Tese de Doutoramento). 2010.

13 Tavares A. Idosos e Atividade Física – programas, qualidade de vida e atitudes. (Tese de Mestrado). 2010.

14 Tribess S, Virtuoso J. Prescrição de Exercícios Físicos para Idosos. Rev Saúde Com. 2005;1(2):163–172.

15 Roubenoff R. Sarcopenia: effects on body composition and function. J Gerontol Med Sci. 2003;58A(11):1012–1017.

16 Roubenoff R, Hughes VA. Sarcopenia: current concepts. J Gerontol A Biol Sci Med Sci. 2000;55(12):M716– M724.

17 Siparsky P, Kirkendall D, Garrett W. Muscle changes in aging: understanding sarcopenia. Sport Heal. 2014;6(1):36–40.

18 Frontera W, Zayas A, Rodriguez N. Aging of human muscle: understanding sarcopenia at the single muscle cell level. Phys Med Rehabil Clin. 2012;23(1):201–207.

19 Frontera WR, Hughes VA, Fielding RA, Fiatarone MA, Evans WJ, Roubenoff R. Aging of skeletal muscle: a 12-yr longitudinal study. J Appl Physiol. 2000;88(4):1321–1326.

20 Narici M V, Maganaris CN, Reeves ND, Capodaglio P. Effect of aging on human muscle architecture. J Appl Physiol. 2003;95(6):2229–2234.

21 Baptista RR, Vaz MA. Arquitetura muscular e envelhecimento: adaptação funcional e aspectos clínicos; revisão da literatura Muscle architecture and aging: functional adaptation and clinical aspects. Lit Rev. 2009;16(4):368–373.

22 Harris-Love M, Monfaredi R, Ismail C, Blackman M, Cleary K. Quantitative ultrasound: measurement considerations for the assessment of muscular dystrophy and sarcopenia. Front Aging Neurosci. 2014;6:1–4.

23 Wilhelm EN, Rech A, Minozzo F, et al. Concurrent strength and endurance training exercise sequence does not affect neuromuscular adaptations in older men. Exp Gerontol. 2014;60:207–214.

24 Narici M V, Maganaris CN. Adaptability of elderly human muscles and tendons to increased loading. J Anat. 2006;208(4):433–443.

25 McNally E. The development and clinical applications of musculoskeletal ultrasound. Skeletal Radiol. 2011;40(9):1223–1231.

26 Santos R. Morphological ultrasound evaluation in acute and chronic muscle overloading. 2017.

27 Delaney S, Worsley P, Warner M, Taylor M, Stokes M. Assessing contractile ability of the quadriceps muscle using ultrasound imaging. Muscle Nerve. 2010;42(4):530–538.

28 Teixeira A. Efeito do treinamento de força na força, espessura muscular e qualidade muscular dos extensores do joelho de homens idosos. 2013.

29 Verhulst F, Leeuwesteijn A, Louwerens J, Geurts A, Van Alfen N, Pillen S. Quantitative ultrasound of lower leg and foot muscles: feasibility and reference values. Foot Ankle Surg. 2011;17(3):145–149.

30 Santos R, Armada-da-silva PAS. Radiography reproducibility of ultrasound-derived muscle thickness and echo-intensity for the entire quadriceps femoris muscle. Radiography. 2017; 23(3):e51–e61.

31 Radaelli R, Neto ENW, Marques MFB, Pinto RS. Espessura e qualidade musculares medidas a partir de ultrassonografia: Influência de diferentes locais de mensuração. Rev Bras Cineantropometria e Desempenho Hum. 2011;13:87–93.

32 Muraki S, Fukumoto K, Fukuda O. Prediction of the muscle strength by the muscle thickness and hardness using ultrasound muscle hardness meter. Springerplus. 2013;2(457):1–7.

33 Wilhelm E, Rech A, Minozzo F, Radaelli R, Botton C, Pinto R. Relationship between quadriceps femoris echo intensity, muscle power, and functional capacity of older men. Age (Omaha). 2014;4:1–6.

34 Santos R, Valamatos MJ, Mil-homens P, Armada-da-silva PAS. Radiography Muscle thickness and echo-intensity changes of the quadriceps femoris muscle during a strength training program. Radiography. 2018; 24(4):e75–e84.

35 Santos L., Parente C., Ribeiro J., Pontes A. Promoção Da Saúde. Vol I. 2015.

36 Direção-Geral da Saúde. "Quem? Eu? exercício?" Exercício sem riscos para lá dos sessenta. In: Autocuidados Na Saúde e Na Doença – Guia Para as Pessoas Idosas. Lisboa: Ministério. 2001:1–45.

37 Alves R, Mota J, Costa C, Guilherme J, Alves B. Physical fitness and elderly health effects of hydrogymnastics. Rev Bras Med Esporte. 2004;10(1):38–43.

38 Gómez-Cabello A, Carnicero J a, Alonso-Bouzón C, et al. Age and gender, two key factors in the associations between physical activity and strength during the ageing process. Maturitas. 2014;78(02):106–112.

39 Miranda A, Picorelli A, Pereira D, et al. Adherence of older women with strength training and aerobic exercise. Clin Interv Aging. 2014;9:323–331.

40 Cadore E, Pinto R, Bottaro M, Izquierdo M. Strength and endurance training prescription in healthy and frail elderly. Aging Dis. 2014;5(1):1–13.

41 Baptista R, Onzi E, Goulart N, Dos Santos L, Makarewicz G, Vaz M. Effects of concentric versus eccentric strength training on the elderly's knee extensor structure and function. J Exerc Physiol Online. 2016;19(3):120–133.

11 Structural and functional changes of the aging heart

Joaquim Castanheira and Telmo Pereira

Introduction

Aging is known to be a dynamic, progressive, and irreversible process closely linked to biological, psychological, and social factors[1,2] and modulated by the environment, lifestyle, and genetic factors.[3] In the *World Population Prospects – The 2015 Revision* report, the United Nations places Portugal on the list of the six fastest aging countries. By the year 2050, about 40% of the Portuguese population will be over 60, a number that is above the European average. In terms of the world population, generational aging will mean an increase from 901 million to 2.1 billion people over 60 in the next three decades, a number that could triple by 2100.[4]

According to the World Health Organization (WHO), cardiovascular diseases are the leading cause of death in the world – 17.5 million people in 2012. Of these, 80% are due to myocardial infarction and stroke. Thus, the adoption of preventive strategies for these major cardiovascular events are a major strategic action in order to avoid the social and economic burden associated with these diseases.[5] Several studies indicate that the susceptibility to the development of chronic morbidities at both structural and functional levels is associated with increased chronological age.[6–9] Although changes in the cardiovascular system can occur in any individual and at any age, the rates at which they occur differ at varying chronological and functional ages. The understanding of the relationship between aging and the inherent cardiac changes is therefore an important requirement for the broader understanding of aging.

The aging heart

Changes in the heart valves

With aging, the most frequent changes observed in the heart concern the structure and function of the valves, particularly the valves

DOI: 10.4324/9781003215271-11

in the left part of the heart. The fibrocalcification of the leaflets and subvalvular apparatus of the mitral valve and calcification and dilation of the aortic root, with subsequent functional consequences are particularly common. Although the right heart valves are not so affected, there is evidence of small fibroelastic nodules in the tricuspid valve, while the pulmonary valve remains mostly unchanged with aging.[10–12] Lambl outgrowths (acellular deposits covered by a single layer of endothelium)[13] are believed to represent a common valvular degenerative change and often appear to reflect the wear and tear of the leaflets. Some authors consider them to represent repetitive trauma-related endothelial proliferations.[14,15] The most frequently found changes in the aortic valve relate to fibrosis and calcification caused by valve tissue wear and tear. The valvular calcification process has much in common with atherosclerosis and bone formation. About 10% of individuals with aortic fibrosclerosis will progress to develop aortic stenosis after a few years.[16] Considering the mitral valve, localized calcification at the ring level is frequent, with the most common site being the base of the posterior leaflet. Calcium extension at the leaflet level is rarer. As the size of the left ventricular cavity decreases with advancing age, the area containing the mitral valve leaflets and the chordae tendineae decreases. Thus, during ventricular systole, the mitral valve leaflets are projected to the left atrium, a movement very similar to the mitral valve prolapse pattern.[17] Incidentally, this decrease in the long axis of the left ventricle and partly the right deviation of the dilated ascending aorta causes an inclination of the interventricular septum to the outflow chamber, which is commonly referred to as the sigmoid interventricular septum.[18]

Changes in heart function

Heart failure affects more than 5% of the population after 60 years of age, 10% between 65 and 75 years and 20% over 80 years. However, at rest, changes associated with systolic volume and cardiac output are insignificant when compared to young individuals,[7,19] favoring the maintenance of a relatively preserved systolic function since contractile responses to beta-adrenergic stimuli decrease with aging.[20] However, authors such as Masugata et al.[20] and others[21] admit that for ages greater than or equal to ninety years, some depression of systolic function may also occur.

Unlike systolic function, diastolic function is closely related to age.[7] Although there may be no compromise in myocardial contractility with aging, the fact is that the ventricular relaxation process is slowed down with an increase in atrial systole's contribution to final diastolic volume and cardiac output through the Frank–Starling mechanism.[7,22,23] With aging, the heart rate, the contractile response to hypotension and to exercise and catecholamines also decrease, due to decreased sensitivity to sympathetic stimuli as a result of decreased beta-receptor stimulation. This "physiological" diastolic dysfunction in the older adult can be explained by the deterioration of the relaxation and of the passive properties of the left ventricular filling.[24,25] Thus, with the use of tissue Doppler echocardiography, it is possible to observe, with advancing age, an inverse correlation of the velocities of the E' and A' waves of the septal and mitral valve. This reflects a gradual decline in the initial left ventricular diastolic filling with a compensatory increase in the contribution of atrial systole in order to maintain an adequate ventricular filling volume.[25]

Arterial changes

As for the major vessels (aorta and pulmonary artery), aging encompasses an increase in arterial stiffness as a result of calcium deposition and loss of elastic fibers of the middle layer, a complex phenomenon characterized by decreased arterial compliance.[26] Clinically, this stiffness may be manifested by an increased pulse pressure and isolated systolic hypertension.[27,28] In particular, aortic stiffening contributes to an increase in systolic blood pressure and a decrease in diastolic blood pressure, which is associated with an increase in left ventricular afterload and a decrease in mean coronary perfusion pressure,[29] which occurs mainly in diastole. Given that there is also a decreased response to stimulation of adrenergic receptors, baroreceptors, and chemoreceptors, and an increase in circulating catecholamines, the onset of systolic arterial hypertension, diastolic dysfunction, and heart failure is stimulated.[7,21,22]

The AGA@4life intervention model

The validation project for the AGA@4life model included the application of M-mode, two-dimensional, classic Doppler, and tissue Doppler modalities on 38 old adults (28 female and 11 male), aged between 65 and 92 years (average 82.5 years). We sought to evaluate the benefits of a personalized and multidisciplinary intervention in the overall health of the older adult, with particular focus on cardiac structure and function.

Regarding the structural and functional changes found in the aortic valve, 84.6% of the individuals (78.8% ♀ and 21% ♂) had fibrosis (although mild fibrosis was predominant: 72.7%) and 48.7% regurgitation (68% ♀ and 26% ♂). Regarding the mitral valve, 64% of the individuals (80% ♀ and 20% ♂) presented fibrosis (discrete fibrosis in 36%) and 64% regurgitation (84% ♀ and 18% ♂). At the tricuspid valve, 28% of individuals had regurgitation (81.8% ♀ and 2.7% ♂) with 5 of the individuals having a pulmonary artery systolic pressure above 35 mmHg. The pulmonary valve showed no significant changes.

Other infrequent structural changes were also found, such as impaired left ventricular contractility, hypertrophy of the basal segment of the interventricular septum, mitral valve annulus calcification, bulging and aneurysmal configuration of the interatrial septum, dilated ascending aorta, very slight posterior pericardial effusion, and one individual with mechanical prosthesis placed in the aortic position.

Cardiac assessment after the implementation of the intervention program, integrating components of adapted physical exercise, nutritional adjustment, pharmacotherapeutic counseling and complementary psychosocial activities, produced significant effects on several functional parameters of the older adult, revealing cardiovascular benefits with potential implications in terms of their ability to perform daily activities with autonomy and the overall quality of life.

Conclusion

The aging of modern societies is one of the great challenges of the approaching decades, and the development of strategies to promote successful aging that guarantee the social participation of the older adult in the various aspects of life is critical.

At the strictly cardiac level, the changes associated with aging are widely known, and the rate at which these changes occur is quite heterogeneous, and potentially reversible through the adoption of healthy lifestyle behaviors, beginning at early stages of the individual's life continuum, and continuing during the period of senescence.

Given the heterogeneity of aging, strategies to promote a biologically fit heart during aging should be based on an integrated, multidisciplinary and personalized framework, as advocated in the AGA@4life intervention model. The preliminary results of this intervention model in several cardiac parameters allow us to aim for significant improvements in aspects that may be determinant for a more autonomous and functionally adapted life, so the translation of this model into geriatric clinical practice is highly recommended.

Key points

- Aging is a heterogeneous process accompanied by structural and functional changes at the heart level.
- Physical activity associated with healthy eating promotes the attenuation of age-related cardiac changes.
- Strategies to promote active and healthy aging should be based on a multidisciplinary, integrated, and personalized structure as recommended in the AGA@4life model.

References

1 Lakatta, EG. So! What's aging? Is cardiovascular aging a disease? J Mol Cell Cardiol. 2015;83:1–13.

2 Litvoc J, Brito FC. Envelhecimento – prevenção e promoção de saúde. São Paulo: Atheneu. 2004; 1–16.

3 Fechine B, Trompieri N. O processo de envelhecimento: as principais alterações que acontecem com o idoso com o passar dos anos. Inter-SciencePlace. 2012.

4 United Nations, Department of Economic and Social Affairs, Population Division. World Population Prospects: The 2015 Revision, Key Findings and Advance Tables. Working Paper No. ESA/P/WP.241. 2015.

5 World Health Organization (WHO). Global Hearts Initiative working together to beat cardiovascular disease. 2016.

6 Feridooni HA, Dibb KM, Howlett, SE. How cardiomyocyte excitation calcium release and contraction become altered with age. J Mol Cell Cardiol. 2015;83:62–72.

7 Wajngarten M. O coração no idoso. J Diagn Cardiol. 2010; 13(43):1–9.

8 Jakovljevic DG. Physical activity and cardiovascular aging: physiological and molecular insights. Exp Gerontol. 2018;109:67–74.

9 Cheng S, Yu H, Chen Y, Chen C, Lien W, Yang P, Hu G. Physical activity and risk of cardiovascular disease among older adults. Int J Gerontol. 2013;7(3):133–36.

10 Keller KM, Howlett SE. Sex differences in the biology and pathology of the aging heart. Can J Cardiol. 2016;32:1065–73.

11 Shioi H, Inuzaka Y. Aging as a substrate of heart failure. J Cardiol. 2012;60:423–8.

12 Júnior LM. O envelhecimento e o coração: as valvas. Ponto de Vista. 2016;18(1):58–9; doi: 10.5327/Z1984-4840201625388.

13 Salcedo EE, Cohen GI, White RD, Davison MB. Cardiac tumors: diagnosis and management. Curr Probl Cardiol. 1992;17:73–137.

14 Marina L, Vladimir T, Eli P, Ruthie S, Ricardo K, et al. Clinical significance and prevalence of valvular strands during routine echo examinations. Eur Heart J Cardiovasc Imaging. 2014;15:1226–30.

15 Mohler ER 3rd, Gannon F, Reynolds C, Zimmerman R, Keane MG, et al. Bone formation and inflammation in cardiac valves. Circulation. 2001;103:1522–8.

16 Sahasakul Y, Edwards WD, Naessens JM, Tajik AJ. Age related changes in aortic and mitral valve thickness: implications for two-dimensional echocardiography based on an autopsy study of 200 normal human hearts. Am J Cardiol. 1988;62:424–30.

17 Ranasinghe I, Cheruvu C, Yiannikas J. Sigmoid Septum (SS): an age-related phenomenon or Sigmoid Hypertrophic Cardiomyopathy (sHCM)? Heart Lung Circulation. 2010;19:53.

18 Oxenham H, Sharpe N. Cardiovascular aging and heart failure. Eur J Heart Fail. 2003;5:427–34.

19 Lakatta EG. Introduction: chronic heart failure in older persons. Heart Fail Rev. 2002;7:5–8.

20 Masugata H, Senda S, Goda F, et al. Cardiac function as assessed by echocardiography in the oldest old ≥90 years of age. Int Heart J. 2007;48(4):497–504.

21 Cheitlin MD. Cardiovascular physiology—changes with aging. Am J Geriatric Cardiol. 2003;12(1):9–13.

22 Hall JE. Tratado de Fisiologia Médica. 12°Edição. Rio de Janeiro: Elsevier Editora Ltda. 2011.

23 Alvis BD, Hughes CG. Physiology considerations in the geriatric patient. Anesthesiol Clin. 2015;33(3):447–56. doi: 10.1016/j.anclin.2015.05.003.

24 Pedone MD, Castro I, Hatem D, Haertel JC, Feier F, Pandolfo F. Changes in the parameters of left ventricular diastolic function according to age on tissue Doppler imaging. Arq Bras Cardiol. 2004;83(6):466–69.

25 Zhang Y, Agnoletti D, Xu Y, Wang JG, Blacher J, Safar ME. Carotid-femoral pulse wave velocity in the elderly. J Hypertens. 2014;32(8):1572–6.

26 Chobanian AV, Bakris GL, Black HR, Cushman WC, Green LA, Izzo JL, Jr, et al. The seventh report of the joint national committee on prevention, detection, evaluation, and treatment of high blood pressure: the JNC 7 report. JAMA. 2003;289(19):2560–72.

27 Dart AM, Kingwell BA. Pulse pressure—a review of mechanisms and clinical relevance. J Am Coll Cardiol. 2001;37(4):975–84.

28 Nichols WW, O' Rourke MF, Vlachopoulos C. McDonald's Blood Flow in Arteries: Theoretical, Experimental and Clinical Principles. 6th ed. Boca Raton, FL: Taylor & Francis Group. 2011.

29 Xu B, Daimon M. Cardiac aging phenomenon and its clinical features by echocardiography. Japan Soc Echocardiogr. 2016;14:139–45. doi: 10.1007/s12574-016-0292-6.

12 Modulators and determinants of arterial aging in the older adult

Tatiana Costa and Telmo Pereira

Introduction

The aging process is a systemic process with particular relevance at the vascular level, and particularly the arteries. This relationship between aging and the arterial system is widely known, as stated in Thomas Sydenham aphorism that a person is as older as his/her arteries. The study of the arterial aging is more relevant, when considering that the main causes of death and morbidity in the modern world (cardiovascular diseases) have as common denominator the arterial system. In that way, the modulation of the arterial aging trajectories should be taken as a fundamental strategy in preventive medicine. The identification of arterial benefits as a result of the AGA@4life-based intervention plan supports its effective usefulness in the promotion of organic health in a geriatric population.

In this chapter, we will approach the concepts of arterial aging and review the effects of life-style intervention plans on the arterial function of the older adult.

Arterial aging

Arterial aging is a fundamental sign of the overall biological aging, and is a major determinant of organ function.[1] In order to understand it, it is necessary to address fundamental morphological and functional aspects of the human vascular system.

The arterial wall is composed of three concentric cellular layers, from the exterior to the interior, by this order: adventitia, tunica media, and intima. Lastly, a mono-cellular layer separates the vascular wall from the lumen, the endothelium. The arterial system subdivides itself into two big groups of arteries: central arteries, which are elastic, rich in elastin and collagen; peripheral arteries, smaller and

DOI: 10.4324/9781003215271-12

mostly constituted by smooth muscle. The central arteries of young individuals are elastic and expand, at each contraction, to accommodate the ejection of the blood to the arterial system.[2] These convert the pulsatile flux, originated by the intermittent contractions of the left ventricle (LV), into a stable blood flow to the periphery, allowing a healthy and continuous oxygenation of the organism. In younger individuals, blood pressure (BP) is largely dependent on the arterial resistance provided by the peripheral arteries. With aging, BP gradually becomes more dependent on arterial stiffness. When LV ejects the blood to the aorta, it generates a pressure wave that, while progressing along the arterial tree, is reflected in ramification points. That way, the pressure waveform is the sum of the component ejected by the LV plus these reflected waves, that, in normal situations reach the heart in diastole. The recoil capacity of central arteries in diastole is also essential to a good coronary perfusion.

Arterial aging is accompanied by structural and functional changes with mechanical and hemodynamic consequences. With age, the vascular system suffers several adaptations, such as structural remodeling, which refers to changes in the lumen and in the circumferential configuration of the vessel, and stiffening, which is related to the reduction of the elastic and mechanical properties of the vessel,[3] mostly in the central arteries, which are, *per se*, more elastic than the peripheral ones. From the histological point of view, these arteries suffer an increase of their collagen content and a reduction in the amount of elastin, accompanied by calcification, degradation of elastin, and formation of collagen covalent connections.[4] These changes, that occur on the media layer, are the result of an established balance between three key-mechanisms:

1 Cyclic stress: reflecting the cardiac cycle and its repercussions at the arterial level, namely the proportion of reflected waves.
2 Arterial reparation mechanisms, that correct the lesions promoted by this mechanical-elastic stress.
3 Injuries to the arterial wall provoked by different agents: high BP, dyslipidemia, diabetes, smoking, oxidative stress, endothelial dysfunction, among others.[5]

The endothelium is a key regulator of the vascular tonus, through the action of vasodilating agents, such as nitric oxide (NO), and vasoconstrictors, as endothelin (which is also a strong pro-coagulator). With age, the performance of the endothelium cells becomes unbalanced, with an increase in the production of endothelin and a decrease in the availability of NO. This process of endothelial dysfunction promotes a pro-coagulating state and promotes smooth muscle growth, besides determining variations in the vascular tonus and thus promoting increases in BP.[4]

All these changes contribute to the decrease of artery compliance. The loss of elastic properties in the central arteries originates both a decrease in the quality of blood ejection and an increase in the pulse wave velocity (PWV), an important and reliable way to measure arterial stiffness.[3] Arterial stiffness, in its turn, and particularly when assessed by PWV, is used to stratify cardiovascular risk according to the recommendations of the European Society of Hypertension, due to its independent relation with the risk of major cardiovascular events.[6]

Arterial hypertension (AH), acknowledged as the most important risk factor to the development of cardiovascular diseases, expresses the changes mediated by aging in a straight way. The presence of AH, isolated or in association with other risk factors, such as smoking, obesity, dyslipidemia, and type 2 diabetes, significantly increases the incidence of cardiovascular diseases,[7] such as stroke, coronary disease, heart failure, and kidney disease. With aging, several mechanisms promote the increase in BP, with a common manifestation in older populations – isolated increase of systolic blood pressure (SBP) with maintenance or even decrease of diastolic blood pressure (DBP). This phenomenon is highly dependent on arterial stiffening, and relates to the effect of early reflected waves.[8] This hemodynamic behavior implies an increase in the pulse pressure (difference between SBP and DBP), that corresponds to a context of arterial hyperpulsatility which aggravates the degradation of elastin fibers and progressively compromises the compliance of central arteries. On the other hand, the decrease of DBP and the earlier return of the reflected wave have a negative impact in the coronary perfusion, leading to a reduction in the perfusion pressure in the coronary tree. This causes a hemodynamic unbalance which, associated with the aging-characteristic atherosclerotic phenomena, predisposes the myocardium to ischemic events. The reduction in the contribution of the aorta to maintain adequate diastolic pressures, and the increase in the afterload caused by the loss of arterial compliance, forces the LV to assume a greater pumping protagonism, increasing the overall cardiac work, increasing oxygen consumption and promoting LV hypertrophy (LVH).[9]

AH and arterial stiffness correlate in a physiopathological continuum, which makes it difficult to fully determinate the causality relation. If, in a way, BP increase acts on a mechanical level and leads to an increase in arterial stiffness and thickness, in another way, the increase in stiffness leads to an increase in PWV, and, because of that, an increase in the reflected waves, leading to higher SBP. In this bi-directional relation, links between arterial stiffness and other clinically relevant BP components can also be found, such as the increase in BP and HR variability, and depression in baroreceptor function, which can lead to orthostatic hypotension. On the other hand, arterial stiffness (which eventually will lead to BP increase), is also accelerated by other mechanisms such as metabolic syndrome and inflammatory and neuro-hormonal disturbances that induce endothelial dysfunction.[5]

Early vascular aging (EVA)

Age-dependent changes in the arteries are expected to occur during normal aging, and can be accelerated due to various mechanical, bio-chemical, or metabolic circumstances. Several repairing mechanisms counter-act these aggressions at the local level[1] to promote a biologically normal arterial aging. When the balance between aggression and repairing mechanisms is not sustained, the rate at which the different manifestations of age occur in the arterial system increases and accelerates, confirming the aphorism that a person is as old as his arteries, so that biology dissociates from chronology, leading to a faster arterial aging trajectory than would be expected by chronological age.

The concept of early vascular aging (EVA) emerges as a way to classify the influence of both internal and external factors that lead to the acceleration of arterial aging. This, still evolving, concept congregates the influence of the several factors that could lead to accelerated aging of the arterial system. Table 12.1 summarizes the

Table 12.1 Determinants of the early vascular aging (EVA)

- Increased arterial stiffness and pulse wave velocity;
- Impaired endothelial function;
- Chronic vascular inflammation;
- Intima media thickness and early atherosclerosis;
- Hemorrhagic disturbances;
- Capillary rarefaction and dysfunctional regulation;
- Shorter telomere length/low telomerase activity;
- Impaired glucose and lipid metabolism;
- Insulin resistance;
- Oxidative stress;
- Arterial calcification;
- Increased deposition of matrix substances;
- Small vessel degeneration in brain and kidney;
- Increased afterload and left ventricular hypertrophy.

characteristics that can be associated with EVA,[10] some of which will be further explored throughout this chapter.

As previously mentioned, structural changes in the arterial wall encompasses functional changes. Following this thought, the concept of Hemodynamic Aging Syndrome was established, which relates the hemodynamic changes that occur with aging with the age-dependent increase in arterial stiffness. This is characterized by changes in central and peripheral BP (isolated systolic AH, increased pulse pressure), increased BP variability, decreased heart rate variability, endothelial dysfunction, and depression of baroreceptor function.[11] All these changes have been linked to arterial stiffness, and are both risk factors and consequences of EVA, therefore, constituting relevant clinical features that should be taken into account in the management of the individual's overall cardiovascular risk.

Regarding cardiac function, increased arterial stiffness and the consequently the early reflected wave, leads to an increased afterload, and consequently, LVH, which in turn contributes to a decrease in diastolic coronary perfusion, particularly over the microcirculation due to the high intra-parietal pressure, and the increase in oxygen consumption. These aspects, associated with early reflected wave and a reduction in DBP, increase myocardial vulnerability to ischemia.

Atherosclerosis is a pathological inflammatory phenomenon that is related to endothelial dysfunction and excess deposition of oxidized lipids. With the exposure to risk factors, atherosclerosis progression is faster and leads to increased thickness and calcification of the artery wall, which also contributes to increased arterial stiffness. The association of atherosclerosis with arteriosclerosis (loss of arterial compliance) is common in the vascular aging process, and synergistic effects are expected between both processes, accentuating the organic consequences of this process in terms of morphological and functional decline.

Several risk factors for atherosclerosis are common to cardiovascular disease in general, highlighting a particular role of genetic regulation of the arterial aging continuum. In this context, two major groups of genetic contributions are distinguished: (1) the genes associated with cell signaling (cell wall adhesion molecules) and (2) genes associated with regulation of vascular structure (cytoskeleton cell membrane and extracellular matrix). On the other hand, there are also genetic protective factors (longevity genes) that slow the progression of atherosclerotic and arteriosclerotic diseases, even in the presence of high cholesterol levels and smoking.[4] Also, telomeres are specialized structures of chromatin, which form the protective cover of the DNA helix. These structures shorten with each cell division until the cell can no longer divide. The presence of shorter telomeres has been demonstrated in individuals with EVA, such that telomeres have been studied as potential genetic biomarkers for the presence of EVA.[1]

Determinants of early vascular aging

The success of arterial aging can be determined by comparing the observed versus expected trend of vascular aging, thus comparing vascular and biological age with chronological age. One major challenge is the definition of the best EVA biomarker, considering the existence of several methodologies that are currently under study, including genetic biomarkers (e.g. telomere length), imaging biomarkers (e.g. intima-media thickness), and structural/functional biomarkers (e.g. PWV). Among these biomarkers, PWV has received the most acceptance, given the robust body of evidence that supports its clinical utility, as well as the recognition of its role in risk stratification, as indicated in the most recent international recommendations.[6] Jani and Rajkumar summarized some technical resources available for assessing arterial aging,[4] including:

- Aortic PWV: PWV is an integrated biomarker that reflects the cumulative effect of various risk factors on the arterial system throughout life. It can be obtained using a variety of technological tools and expresses the speed at which the pulse wave travels at a certain arterial distance. The most valid form of assessment is carotid-femoral PWV, which translates to aortic stiffness. PWV is dependent on the viscoelastic properties of the arterial wall and the blood viscosity. The increase in PWV reflects three potential risk factors: increased SBP, increased pulse pressure, and modification of arterial wall properties that cause increased arterial stiffness.
- Augmentation Index (AI): integrated index that allows the estimation of the proportion of the pulse wave that is a consequence of the reflected wave. This coefficient is dependent on PWV and BP and is inversely proportional to heart rate and height.
- Systemic arterial compliance (SAC): This is achieved by simultaneous recording of the ascending aortic blood flow with a Doppler transducer applied on the suprasternal notch and the PPV of the right carotid artery by applanation tonometry. Arterial compliance is then obtained by the formula proposed by Liu et al.[12] which uses the aortic valve measurement obtained by two-dimensional echocardiography.

- Echo-tracking: The use of vascular ultrasound allows the study of local properties of the arteries, measuring the separation of the anterior and posterior walls of a given artery during the systolic cycle, and allowing the determination of the intima-media thickness, an early marker of atherosclerosis.

Determinant factors for accelerated aging vary in different populations, and are strongly related to different lifestyles, particularly in terms of nutritional profile, smoking and level of physical activity, factors known to be associated with increased arterial stiffness.[7] By identifying the factors that lead to early aging in the AGA@4Life project population, we were able to set goals in order to understand the influence of the intervention program on these individuals. In the AGA@4life project cohort, the following factors were identified as determinants of EVA (unpublished data):

- Arterial hypertension: Abnormal PWV values were significantly related to AH (dichotomized variable). Increasing central and peripheral BP values were significantly and independently related to higher PWV values;
- Increased vascular resistances: Individuals with abnormal PWV values had increased vascular resistance, with a linear relationship between the vascular resistance index and PWV;
- Augmentation index: The values of this coefficient correlated linearly with the PWV, as expected;
- Frailty: A linear regression determined an inverse relationship between handgrip strength and PWV, indicating that arterial stiffness and frailty are directly related, and that the presence of EVA translates a globally unfavorable organic context at functional and physiological level;
- Renal function: An association between arterial stiffness and increased creatinine values was obtained, indicating the existence of worse renal function for increasing PWV values, and consequently, the presence of EVA was accompanied by an overall more unfavorable clinical profile.

Positive modulators of the arterial function in the older adult – Role of the AGA@4life intervention model

Regarding arterial aging, prevention should be the cornerstone to promote a more biologically favorable trajectory. The different approaches should be tailored according to the individual's needs, even though two main clusters should be considered as a starting point: (1) older adult with installed risk factors (AH, dyslipidemia, and/or diabetes) and (2) older adult without major risk factors. This difference translates the coexistence of pharmacological therapy on top of non-pharmacological intervention strategies. The non-pharmacological strategies may include lifestyle changes, mainly in the form of adapted physical activity, reduction in salt intake, caloric restriction, reduced alcohol consumption, and smoking cessation. These measures could contribute to BP regulation, weight control, metabolic syndrome prevention, and chronic inflammatory disease control. Additionally, cognitive stimulation programs may help to counteract the cognitive decline associated with aging. In individuals with risk factors under pharmacological treatment, the establishment and maintenance of thorough control and surveillance is essential, as well as the promotion of therapy compliance through counseling, taking into account the therapeutic complexity and the non-pharmacological strategies.

The major benefits of the AGA@4life model in promoting healthy arterial aging mainly resulted from physical activity and nutritional optimization. Sedentary lifestyle is classically associated with AH, obesity, and other metabolic changes, resulting in an accelerated trajectory of arterial stiffness with age. The implementation of adapted physical exercise plans contribute to improved arterial function and mechanics, as previously shown in other studies, in which exercise had a beneficial impact, not only on BP, but also in terms of arterial stiffness, with significant decrease in PWV, and improvement of endothelial function and baroreceptor function.[13]

In terms of nutrition, it is known that salt consumption is closely linked to the development of AH,[14] and has been associated with a higher risk of cerebrovascular events.[15] The implementation of a balanced diet with reduced salt intake for at least 4 weeks has been shown to be associated with a reduction in BP, regardless of gender, ethnicity, and baseline BP levels.[14] A calorie-restricted diet lowers the percentage of cholesterol. The stimulation of regular fluid consumption leads to a more constant volume of circulating blood, and therefore less BP variability. Adequate water consumption may also have a positive impact on baroreceptor function, thus reducing the risk of orthostatic hypotension.[16] The combination of these two components may lead to an additional benefit, weight loss, as obesity is a risk factor for AH and is proven to be associated with PWV.[17]

Cognitive stimulation and sensitization, may lead to increased adherence to therapy, which is essential in hypertensive individuals or those with risk factors for cardiovascular disease such as diabetes or dyslipidemia.

Conclusions

As life expectancy is increasing, major attention should be put on arterial function, and to the identification of individual arterial aging trajectories in which the EVA concept comes in play. It is important that the number of years lived is accompanied by the best possible quality of life. It is imperative to detect and intervene in order to reduce exposure to modifiable risk factors for cardiovascular disease, which are also crucial in early arterial aging.

In older populations, a comprehensive geriatric approach may be a useful and effective strategy for promoting cardiovascular health, given its holistic, multidisciplinary, and personalized nature. Promoting healthy lifestyles through personalized and continuous follow-up, as advocated in the AGA@4life intervention model, may contribute to the readjustment of individual trajectories of arterial aging to biologically more favorable ones, with positive effects in terms of mortality and morbidity reduction. In fact, the preliminary results regarding the implementation of the AGA@4life program identified, as expected, significant improvements in the cardio-vascular health of the older adult cohort, with equally important consequences in terms of quality of life and overall perception of well-being.

A major challenge for the upcoming years will be the translation of this approach into a nationwide program, based on multidisciplinary teams, aimed at implementing this intervention model in a comprehensive and systematic manner, preferentially anchored in primary care units, working in proximity with the older population and in their daily life ecosystem.

Key points

- Arterial stiffening is the most common translation of arterial aging.
- EVA is associated with a worse overall cardiovascular risk profile.
- The implementation of strategies to prevent or promote a good arterial function should be assumed as a strategic priority.
- The intervention programs aimed at correcting EVA should be personalized, multidisciplinary, and systematic.
- The AGA@4life model is an effective non-pharmacological tool for promoting a healthy arterial aging.

References

1 Nilsson PM, Boutouyrie P, Cunha P, Kotsis V, Narkiewicz K, Parati G, Rietzschel E, Scuteri A, Laurent S. Early vascular ageing in translation: from laboratory investigations to clinical applications in cardiovascular prevention. J Hypertens. 2013;31(8):1517–26.

2 Mackey RH, Sutton-Tyrrell K, Vaitkevicius PV, Sakkinen PA, Lyles MF, Spurgeon HA, Lakatta EG, Kuller LH. Correlates of aortic stiffness in elderly individuals: a subgroup of the Cardiovascular Health Study. Am J Hypertens. 2002;15(1 Pt1):16–23.

3 Kohn JC, Lampi MC, Reinhart-King CA. Age-related vascular stiffening: causes and consequences. Front Genet. 2015;6:112.

4 Jani B, Rajkumar C. Ageing and vascular ageing. Postgrad Med J. 2006;82(968):357–62.

5 Cunha PG, Boutouyrie P, Nilsson PM, Laurent S. Early vascular ageing (EVA): definitions and clinical applicability. Curr Hypertens Rev. 2017;13(1):8–15.

6 Williams B, Mancia G, Spiering W, et al. 2018 ESC/ESH guidelines for the management of arterial hypertension. Eur Heart J. 2018;39(33):3021–3104. doi:10.1093/eurheartj/ehy339.

7 Mikael LR, Paiva AMG, Gomes MM, Sousa ALL, Jardim PCBV, Vitorino PVO, Euzébio MB, Sousa WM, Barroso WKS. Vascular aging and arterial stiffness. Arq Bras Cardiol. 2017;109(3):253–8.

8 Laurent S, Cockcroft J, Van Bortel L, Boutouyrie P, Giannattasio C, Hayoz D, Pannier B, Vlachopoulos C, Wilkinson I, Struijker-Boudier H, European Network for Non-invasive Investigation of Large Arteries. Expert consensus document on arterial stiffness: methodological issues and clinical applications. Eur Heart J. 2006;27(21):2588–605.

9 Veerasamy M, Ford GA, Neely D, Bagnall A, MacGowan G, Das R, Kunadian V. Association of aging, arterial stiffness, and cardiovascular disease: a review. Cardiol Rev. 2014;22(5):223–32

10 Nilsson PM. Early vascular aging (EVA): consequences and prevention. Vasc Health Risk Manag. 2008;4(3):547–52.

11 Nilsson PM. Hemodynamic aging as the consequence of structural changes associated with early vascular aging (EVA). Aging Dis. 2014;5(2):109–13.

12 Liu Z, Brin KP, Yin FC. Estimation of total arterial compliance: an improved method and evaluation of current methods. Am J Physiol. 1986;251(3 Pt2):H588–600.

13 Cameron JD, Rajkumar C, Kingwell BA, Jennings GL, Dart AM. Higher systemic arterial compliance is associated with greater exercise time and lower blood pressure in a young older population. J Am Geriatr Soc. 1999;47(6):653–6.

14 He FJ, Li J, Macgregor GA. Effect of longer-term modest salt reduction on blood pressure. Cochrane Database Syst Rev. 2013;(4):CD004937.

15 Strazzullo P, D'Elia L, Kandala NB, Cappuccio FP. Salt intake, stroke, and cardiovascular disease: meta-analysis of prospective studies. BMJ. 2009;339:b4567.

16 Shannon JR, Diedrich A, Biaggioni I, Tank J, Robertson RM, Robertson D, Jordan J. Water drinking as a treatment for orthostatic syndromes. Am J Med. 2002;112(5):355–60.

17 Petersen KS, Blanch N, Keogh JB, Clifton PM. Effect of weight loss on pulse wave velocity: systematic review and meta-analysis. Arterioscler Thromb Vasc Biol. 2015;35(1):243–52.

13 Hepatic characterization of the senior population and its relationship with polymedication

Rute Santos

Introduction

Associated with an aging population, changing habits often leads to the acceleration of the process and factors that are inherent to it. It is important to raise awareness of the older population and their caregivers and family members to promote changes in attitudes and behaviors that benefit the aging process, easing it into a slower and healthier continuum. In order to achieve it, the use of intervention strategies and programs is crucial, making individuals conscientious, responsible, and enhancers of their own health. These initiatives involve not only the promotion of physical activity but also the change in food habits and medication adherence and a knowledgeable and controlled intake.

The aging process

Aging is often associated with decreased health and quality of life[1–3]. Human aging involves the transformation of all processes, physical, psychological, and social, with implication on the social participation of the individual[3]. Thus, aging can be considered a dynamic and progressive process, in which there are morphological, functional, and biochemical changes and that depends on each individual, leading to individual and group differences regarding rhythm, duration, and effects of this process. These changes are age-dependent, event-dependent and have interaction links including genetic-biological and socio-historical-psychological[1]. Many changes occur with aging, particularly, decreased efficiency of the cardiovascular system, less elastic cartilage, lower muscle strength, coordination loss, onset of osteoporosis, muscle mass loss, slower digestive system, decreased efficiency of urinary and glandular systems, among others. Considering

DOI: 10.4324/9781003215271-13

all these factors, biological and functional age becomes the most appropriate way to measure aging and its adaptations[1,3].

Aging and liver changes

Aging is characterized by a progressive decline in cellular functions although the aged liver seems to preserve its function relatively well. However, morphological changes in the liver are expected to occur with aging, such as decreased size due to a lower hepatic blood flow[4]. Diet is considered a main environmental determinant of the life span and aging trajectories. It also has a major impact on liver aging, the central metabolic organ of the body. Drug therapy in the older adult can be complicated by several factors, such as declining body weight, renal function, liver mass, and hepatic blood flow, making adverse drug reactions more frequent. Antihypertensive therapy in the older adult depends on liver or renal function and should be adjusted accordingly[4,5].

Aging is also associated with declining intrinsic metabolic activity of the liver parenchyma and gene expression of proteins involved in intermediate metabolism, mitochondrial respiration and drug metabolism. Aged hepatocytes accumulate oxidative DNA damage, responsible for the increase of mutations, particularly in the mitochondrial genome[6,7].

Aging and polymedication

Underlying aging is the appearance of potentially drug-treated co-morbidities, so the concept of polymedication emerges, which is defined as the simultaneous use of 5 or more medications for more than 3 months, or the excessive administration of non-prescribed and non-needed drugs[8]. Hence, the association of several pharmacological therapies is common in the old adult, each for a specific health need. However, it is important to understand if the benefits outweigh the harms of this multi-medication as they may change over time. That is, it becomes important to understand whether or not a drug provides substantial benefit according to individual goals and needs, whether or not the risk of side effects increases, and whether the harm of a drug outweighs the benefits.

On the other hand, the risk of side effects increases with more medications as well as increasing age. A recent, well-conducted systematic review showed that adverse drug effects occur in 58% of people taking five drugs[9]. Older people are especially susceptible to the adverse effects of medications, and are also prone to non-compliance to the prescribed treatment as a result of the therapeutic complexity and/or its side effects.

It is important to take into account that any type of medication affects the body, and that both processes are fundamental to understand the benefits and harms of polymedication[8,9]. One of the most important concerns when taking multiple medications is the risk of interactions. These interactions may increase the effect of the drug on the body or diminish its effect, that is, some combined drugs may produce a "new effect" or interaction that may be helpful or harmful[9]. On the other hand, when the medicine enters the body it goes through a series of metabolic processing steps. These processes consist of absorption, distribution to different parts of the body, depending on their properties – metabolism that usually occurs in the liver – and elimination[8].

With aging, changes occur in the way the body processes drugs and the benefit/risk profile of a drug may change. Polymedication can become a problem if medications (and vitamins, herbs, and other dietary supplements) interact to increase, decrease, or cancel the effects of each other[8,9]. Therefore, it is essential to prescribe medication to the older adult with special attention, as complications associated with medication are common (e.g. adverse reactions and drug interactions). Pharmacological knowledge is essential, as this is the only way to identify and prescribe different drugs properly and to advise their safe, correct and effective use. A balance must be found between disease treatment and adverse effects reduction in order to optimize drug use[8,9]. On the other hand, adherence to pharmacological therapy is also important, which consists in how the older person follows the instructions given by the health professionals regarding the prescribed medication(s), and perform it correctly. Non-adherence to therapy is known to be highly prevalent in geriatric patients and has been related to several factors such as the number of medications taken, difficulty in swallowing, denial of illness, psychological problems, dementia, economic difficulties, socio-cultural, and self-medication[10].

Hepatic impairment

The liver is the only internal human organ capable of naturally regenerating lost tissue. The aging process predisposes to functional and structural hepatic impairment and metabolic risk[6]. Steatosis is a liver disease characterized by high accumulation of fats such as triglycerides in the liver, totaling more than 10% of the total weight of this organ[11]. About one third of the western adult population is estimated to have some degree of steatosis and its incidence is expected to increase, as is the incidence of obesity and type II diabetes[12].

This condition has been associated with several causes that include viruses such as hepatitis B and C, alcohol consumption, smoking habits, polymedication, idiopathic causes, obesity and diabetes, all of which may contribute to an increase in liver size[11,13,14].

Steatosis is a pathological liver condition that is generally difficult to characterize and detect due to its sometimes disguised characteristics or its mimicry with other pathologies[13,15]. It is typically a symptomatically silent and reversible pathology, but may evolve into more complex situations such as cirrhosis or hepatocellular carcinoma[13,16].

Ultrasound as a method of liver evaluation

The evacuation of the liver has been facilitated by the technological evolution that began some decades ago, especially in the field of imaging, which created instrumentation to aid the visual capacity of health professionals and consequently provided a preferential tool to diagnose and monitor liver pathological conditions[17,18].

Biopsy, despite being the gold standard method for detecting liver pathologies, has some drawbacks such as its invasive character and the uncertainty regarding the sampling tissue area[19–21]. These disadvantages have led to the adoption of new methods, which include imaging techniques that are being used increasingly in clinical practice[21,22].

Technological advances and several ultrasound advantages such as low-cost, patient-tolerability, non-invasiveness, non-ionizing radiation technique, high sensitivity and specificity, makes abdominal ultrasonography a reliable method for qualitative and even quantitative evaluation of hepatic morphological changes. Ultrasound can most often characterize the structures regarding their echogenicity, echo-structure, contours and dimensions, and pathologies such as malignant or benign nodules can be detected[23].

In current hospital practice, the difference in eco-intensity between two structures is made qualitatively and is dependent on the visual perception of the health professional. The adoption of quantitative analysis is expected to be associated with greater efficacy and better diagnostic performance[11,13,24].

On the other hand, the kidney, as a closer structure to the liver, is considered a reference in the morphological evaluation of the liver, since its echo intensity is similar to the one found in liver parenchyma. The kidney is the organ chosen as a reference for comparison because its identification is easy and its proximity to the liver allows images of the two organs to be obtained. Typically, there is an increase in liver echogenicity (it becomes more reflective) relative to the renal cortex in cases of steatosis[24], making a qualitative assessment of its morphology possible. However, small adipose infiltrations in the liver parenchyma may go unnoticed in a qualitative approach, making a more detailed assessment of eco-intensity necessary[11,14,24]. Based on the calculation of the difference between liver and kidney echogenicity densities (hepatorenal coefficient), liver echogenicity is measured. When kidney echogenicity is used for comparison, hepatic steatosis is recognized by a brilliant echogenicity pattern (hyper-echogenicity). This method has a specificity and sensitivity of approximately 93% and 89%, respectively[24,25].

Liver steatosis, aging, and polymedication

The articulation of these three concepts leads to a simple sequence of reasoning: with aging, the liver experiences detrimental morphological and functional changes that can be enhanced by polymedication. Hence, it is expected that a polymedicated older adult will present abnormalities in the liver ultrasonography, namely in the echogenicity parameters, showing a hyper-echo-intensity when compared to the kidney.

In the initial evaluation and characterization of the older population who underwent the AGA@4life intervention program, hepatic steatosis was found in most of the 54 participants included, showing a high hepatorenal index. In association, the nutritional profile was found to be worst in those participants with abnormal liver results. Expectedly, polymedicated participants were also amongst the ones with liver abnormalities. These results are in line with the literature, which shows hepatic abnormalities in the older adult, particularly when polymedication is present[4,8,9,13,23,26,27].

AGA@4life intervention program: beneficial effect of pharmacological counseling on hepatic steatosis

One of the goals of the AGA@4life program is to advise healthy lifestyles regarding physical activity, fall prevention, nutritional optimization, cognitive stimulation, psychosocial wellbeing, and pharmacological counseling. As mentioned earlier, polymedication is a common finding in the old adult. Changing habits with regard to polymedication may lead to positive changes, namely in terms of liver morphology. Preliminary results of hepatic ultrasound assessment showed differences in individual participants 3 months after the pharmacological advice, even though the group effect failed to reach the significance criterion. In some cases, the hepatorenal index markedly decreased after the intervention. Of course, it is important to bear in mind that this same intervention program also addressed food issues that may also contribute to the improvement of liver characterization. There are several studies that corroborate these preliminary results, although major changes are expected to occur in the long term population[4,9,26,27].

Conclusions

Aging is characterized by a wide range of biological, functional, and physical changes with consequences in terms of the autonomy, social participation and overall quality of life. Therefore, intervention programs focused on the individual needs and aimed at promoting healthy lifestyles and behavioral changes are essential to prevent major complications and promote favorable aging trajectories. The results observed under the AGA@4life scope, although preliminary, reinforce the need to promote strategies and intervention programs to slow down the aging process, to improve the quality of life, converging on each individual and his daily life ecosystem. The proper pharmacological management of the old adult, hand-in-hand with appropriated nutritional planes is an essential strategic axis to protect the liver through the lifespan.

Key points

- Aging is unavoidable, however, it is up to each individual to slow this process and ensure the best possible quality of life through the lifespan.
- The population's awareness for changing habits regarding disease prevention and health promotion is the cornerstone of the whole process of improving the quality of life and mitigating the aging process.

References

1 Marinho M, Pasqualotti A, Lucia E, Mara L. Envelhecimento humano e as alterações na postura corporal do idoso. Rev Bras Ciências da Saúde. 2010;8(26):52–58.
2 Narici M V, Maganaris CN, Reeves ND, Capodaglio P. Effect of aging on human muscle architecture. J Appl Physiol. 2003;95(6):2229–2234.

3 Santos R. Programa de Intervenção em idosos: atividade física, autonomia funcional e qualidade de vida Programa de Intervenção em idosos: atividade física, autonomia funcional e qualidade de vida. 2014.

4 Tajiri K, Shimizu Y. Liver physiology and liver diseases in the elderly. World J Gastroenterol. 2013;19(46):8459–8467.

5 Golchin N, Frank SH, Vince A, Isham L, Meropol SB. Polypharmacy in the elderly. J Res Pharm Pract. 2015;4(2):85–88.

6 Sheedfar F, Biase S Di, Koonen D, Vinciguerra M. Liver diseases and aging: friends or foes? Aging Cell. 2013;12:950–954.

7 Cieslak KP, Baur O, Verheij J, Bennink RJ, Gulik TM Van. Liver function declines with increased age. Int Hepato-Pancreato-Biliary Assoc. 2016;18(8):691–696.

8 Mclachlan AJ, Pont LG. Drug metabolism in older people—a key consideration in achieving optimal outcomes with medicines. J Gerontol Biol Sci. 2012;67A(2):175–180.

9 Nobili A, Garattini S, Mannucci PM. Multiple diseases and polypharmacy in the elderly: challenges for the internist of the third millennium. J Comorb. 2011;1:28–44.

10 Yap AF, Hons P, Thirumoorthy T, London F, Kwan YH, Hons P. Medication adherence in the elderly. J Clin Gerontol Geriatics. 2016;7(2):64–67.

11 Marshall RH, Eissa M, Bluth EI, Gulotta PM, Davis NK. Hepatorenal index as an accurate, simple, and effective tool in screening for steatosis. Am J Roentgenol. 2012;199(5):997–1002.

12 Bedogni G, Miglioli L, Masutti F, Tiribelli C, Marchesini G, Bellentani S. Prevalence of and risk factors for nonalcoholic fatty liver disease: the Dionysos nutrition and liver study. Hepatology. 2005;42(1):44–52.

13 Lee MJ, Bagci P, Kong J, et al. Liver steatosis assessment: correlations among pathology, radiology, clinical data and automated image analysis software. Pathol Res Pract. 2013;209(6):371–379.

14 Park SK, Seo MH, Shin HC, Ryoo JH. Clinical availability of nonalcoholic fatty liver disease as an early predictor of type 2 diabetes mellitus in Korean men: 5-year prospective cohort study. Hepatology. 2013;57(4):1378–1383.

15 Tarantino G, Costantini S, Finelli C, et al. Carotid intima-media thickness is predicted by combined eotaxin levels and severity of hepatic steatosis at ultrasonography in obese patients with nonalcoholic Fatty liver disease. PLoS One. 2014;9(9):e105610.

16 Krishnan A, Venkataraman J. Prevalence of nonalcoholic fatty liver disease and its biochemical predictors in patients with type-2 diabetic mellitus. Exp Clin Hepatol. 2011;7(3–4):7–10.

17 Santos AA. Classificação Da Esteatose Hepática Usando Imagens Ecográficas. Faculdade de Ciências e Tecnologia da Universidade de Coimbra, Coimbra, Portugal; 2012.

18 Pereira AS, Rafael JA. Processamento de imagem em medicina. Acta Med Port. 1992;5(1):23–27.

19 Hernaez R, Lazo M, Bonekamp S, et al. Diagnostic accuracy and reliability of ultrasonography for the detection of fatty liver: a meta-analysis. Hepatology. 2011;54(3):1082–1090.

20 Lewis JR, Mohanty SR. Nonalcoholic fatty liver disease: a review and update. Dig Dis Sci. 2010;55(3):560–578.

21 Brunt EM, Tiniakos DG. Histopathology of nonalcoholic fatty liver disease. World J Gastroenterol. 2010;16(42):5286–5296.

22 Dumitrascu DL, Neuman MG. Non-alcoholic fatty liver disease: an update on diagnosis. Clujul Med. 2018;91(2):147–150.

23 Wang J-H, Hung C-H, Kuo F-Y, et al. Ultrasonographic quantification of hepatic-renal echogenicity difference in hepatic steatosis diagnosis. Dig Dis Sci. 2013;58(10):2993–3000.

24 Syakalima M, Takiguchi M, Yasuda J, et al. Comparison of attenuation and liver–kidney contrast of liver ultrasonographs with histology and biochemistry in dogs with experimentally induced steroid hepatopathy. Vet Q. 1998;20(1):18–22.

25 von Volkmann HL, Havre RF, Løberg EM, et al. Quantitative measurement of ultrasound attenuation and hepato-renal index in non-alcoholic fatty liver disease. Med Ultrason. 2013;15(1):16–22.

26 Bertolotti M, Lonardo A, Mussi C, Baldelli E. Nonalcoholic fatty liver disease and aging: epidemiology to management. World J Gastroenterol. 2014;20(39):14185–14204.

27 Gagliano N, Annoni G. Mechanisms of aging and liver functions. Dig Dis. 2007;25:118–123.

14 Cognitive function and aging

Telmo Pereira

Introduction

The proportion of people over 65 years of age has been increasing world-wide[1]. In fact, the aging rate (number of people over 60 per 100 children under 15) is increasing, and it is estimated that by 2025 over 20% of the European population will be over 65 years[2,3]. This population concept of demographic aging, that is, increasing proportion of older people in the total population, is intrinsically associated with the individual process of biological aging, which can be defined as a progressive path of deterioration of physiological functions, with a gradual increase in vulnerability of the organism to disease and increased risk of death[2].

The impact of aging on cognitive function is particularly relevant, so it is of utmost importance to understand thoroughly the processes that mediate the loss of cognitive function with aging, both in the process of normal senescence and in the processes of pathological aging. In fact, population aging will be accompanied by an increase in the varying degrees of reduced cognitive skills, ranging from milder forms of commitment to deeper dementias. The impact of cognitive impairment on the daily life of the older adult, and in their ability to live in an autonomous and socially adjusted manner, make it imperative to identify cognitive preservation strategies that optimize or correct the biological trajectory of functional loss, ensuring health and well-being. In this chapter, we will review the neurocognitive changes that convoy with aging and the possible strategies to promote better cognitive function in the older person.

The aging brain

Neuroscientific research has significantly contributed to the under-standing of the morphological and functional changes of the brain associated with the aging of the human organism. This, in turn,

DOI: 10.4324/9781003215271-14

establishes the fundamental bases for understanding the neuro-cognitive changes identified in the aging process. One aspect that has been identified is the progressive reduction in gray matter volume, with particular prominence in the prefrontal cortex[4,5], and more moderately in the temporal lobe, with particular expression in the hippocampus[6]. The mechanisms involved are diverse and may include neuronal death, neuronal size reduction, and synaptic density reduction[7,8,9]. It is recognized that neurons undergo morphological changes with aging, which include decreased dendritic afforestation and size, and decreased dendritic spines[10]. The reduction of specific subclasses of dendritic spines in the dorsolateral prefrontal cortex has been associated with the impairment of working memory in primates[11], adding arguments to support the hypothesis of a synaptic plasticity compromise as a key element of cognitive impairment associated with aging. Neuronal aging in the hippocampus and prefrontal cortex is also associated with disturbances in calcium homeostasis and electrophysiological modifications that increase the time required for neuronal repolarization, coinciding with a reduction in the levels of neurotrophic factors such as BDNF (brain derived neurotrophic factor)[12]. The deterioration in communication between neurons may also be due to a deregulation in the genes responsible for synaptic protein synthesis[13], related to the occurrence of inflammatory processes and oxidative stress during the later stages in life[14].

In association with synaptic changes, there is also evidence supporting the coexistence of aging-dependent changes in neurotransmitter functioning and bioavailability. In fact, AMPA (α-amino-3-hydroxy-5-methyl-4-isoxazolepropionic acid) receptors, particularly involved in processes such as memory, learning, and synaptic plasticity, have been identified as an important element in the aging process, with evidence of a reduction in the number of these receptors with advancing age[15]. On the other hand, the reduction in neurotransmitter production has also been reported, with important implications for the several dependent cognitive processes[16].

Another explanatory aspect for gray matter volume loss is the accumulation of beta-amyloid protein, which is very prominent in patients with Alzheimer's dementia, but is also present in the older adult with moderate cognitive impairment[17]. Recent studies have shown that the accumulation of this protein in cognitively normal people is associated with an increased risk of developing cognitive impairment over time[18]. In addition, white matter suffers a reduction in volume with aging, of much greater magnitude than that observed in gray matter[19]. Loss of white matter volume may reach 16% to 20% in people over 70 years of age[20], leading to a reduction in the communication of the various interhemispheric brain circuits and a compromise in the communication with the hippocampus, anticipating the occurrence of a decline in cognitive processes such as memory[20,21]. In addition to this structural compromise, aging also conditions functional loss in white matter, disturbing normal neuronal signaling and, consequently, contributing to the occurrence of cognitive decline with advancing age. Other modifications are summarized in Table 14.1.

Cognitive function and aging

The occurrence of changes in cognitive processes is one of the most noticeable manifestations of the aging process, occurring along heterogeneous trajectories of functional decline, whose impact on daily activities will depend on the degree of commitment. When framed in a so-called normal aging, cognitive impairment usually does not limit the ability of the older adult to perform their activities effectively and independently.

Processing speed

Processing speed reflects the efficiency of cognitive processes, that is, the speed with which cognitive activities and motor responses are performed. Its reduction is a characteristic of aging, beginning around the third decade of life and extending throughout life[22]. This reduction can compromise performance in other cognitive domains, such as memory and language, and have a negative influence on social skills that depend on one's ability to communicate and interact with others.

Memory

Another cognitive dimension commonly affected in older people is memory. First, because the acquisition rate (ability to encode new information in memory) gradually decreases with aging[23], as does the

Table 14.1 Additional changes in the aging brain

Neuronal and microglia senescence
Reduction of neuronal plasticity
Cytoskeletal Modifications
Changes in the quantity and distribution of neurotransmitters

ability to access recent information. However, the retention of effectively processed information is cognitively preserved in healthy older adult, but not in dementia[24]. Episodic (or autobiographical) memory is progressively reduced throughout life while the decline in semantic memory usually occurs at a later age[25]. These two forms of memory integrate the declarative (explicit) memory, which corresponds to the ability to recall/remember consciously facts and events. The non-declarative (or implicit) memory remains unchanged throughout life[26]. The decline in memory may further express slower processing, less recourse to learning and memory optimization strategies, difficulty concentrating, increasing distraction from irrelevant information, aspects that collectively contribute to a progressive decline in immediate and short-term memory[27,28]. Working memory, on the other hand, refers to the ability to hold temporarily available information in the mind while it is being processed or used, and is a key element in other cognitive abilities such as problem solving and decision-making. Several studies have documented its decline with aging, particularly when framed in more complex tasks[29].

Attention

The ability to concentrate and focus on a specific stimulus and to process relevant information, or attention, also changes with aging, particularly with regard to complex attention tasks such as selective attention (ability to focus attention on relevant information while ignoring contextual irrelevant information) or divided attention (ability to direct attention to several tasks simultaneously)[29,30]. For sustained attention, that is, the ability to maintain concentration on a task over a long period of time, some evidence has suggested its preservation in a context of healthy aging[31,32].

Executive functions

Executive functions encompass a set of cognitive resources and skills that enable a person to have contextually adjusted behaviors, including the notion of autonomy, independence, and purpose in decision-making. Cognitive resources included in executive functions include aspects such as planning, organization, reasoning, mental flexibility and strategic sense, and the ability to solve problems, adapt to new situations, and adjust behavior during social interaction. In this sense, some studies have shown a decline in some of these aspects with aging, namely in terms of mental flexibility, capacity for abstraction and conceptual formation[33]. This decline can affect an individual's ability to make appropriate decisions and inhibit behavioral responses, and is related to an impaired performance of instrumental daily activities.

Also, the reasoning capacity presents an age-dependent decline. This ability refers to logical thinking in the processes of decision-making and problem-solving. The decline in this capacity occurs in both deductive and inductive reasoning, following a roughly linear path.

Language

Despite being a complex cognitive dimension, language skills tend to remain preserved throughout life, and there may be an enrichment, for example, in the level of vocabulary richness and diversity[34]. However, some studies have shown a decline in verbal fluency with aging[33].

Visuospatial capacity

Understanding space in two and three dimensions involves a set of cognitive resources that change with aging, particularly with regard to the ability to visually construct, that is, the ability to associate individual parts to construct a coherent whole. Aspects such as the perception of objects, the recognition of familiarity, the spatial perception, and the aesthetic notion tend to be preserved in a context of normal aging, being compromised in dementia situations.

Note that the cognitive changes identified with aging coincide with cellular and molecular modifications, expressing a morpho-functional continuum that has been well documented in humans and animal research. Age-dependent deterioration of the prefrontal cortex and the hippocampus, in particular, has been largely associated with cognitive decline in aging. For example, the hippocampus and prefrontal cortex are both deeply linked to memory[35], while the prefrontal cortex is also deeply implicated in high-level cognitive skills and executive functions[36].

Study of cognitive function in the older adult

There are currently several instruments for measuring cognitive function, although controversy still exists in identifying the best instrument or test for each cognitive dimension or population to be analyzed. Examples of instruments applied in the study of cognition of the older adult include the Montreal Cognitive Assessment Battery (MOCA), the Mini-Mental State Examination, or the Telephone Interview for Cognitive Status. Other more sophisticated alternatives involve the use of digital resources with implementation of interactive games and measurement of cognitive performance. One of the platforms currently available, and widely used in the study of cognition associated with aging and dementia, is the Cambridge Neuropsychological Test Automated Battery (CANTAB – Cambridge Cognition, Cambridge, UK)[37,38], which allows for the evaluation of different dimensions of cognitive performance, such as memory, processing speed, attention, executive functions, learning, among others. This platform works in a digital environment, operated through a tablet (touchscreen) and controlled by dedicated software, allowing individual monitoring with evaluation of the functional trajectories and the effect of any interventions in an individual plan, thus allowing for personalized adjustments of on-going intervention programs. The CANTAB offers a wide range of widely validated cognitive tests such as the Motor Screening Task (MOT), the Reaction Time (RTI), the Paired Associates Learning (PAL), the Spatial Working Memory (SWM) and the Rapid Visual Information Processing. Taken together, these tests provide indicators of Attention, Processing Speed, Episodic Memory, Working Memory, and Learning, with additional indicators for flexibility and strategy.

Variability of the cognitive function decline in the older adult

Since cognitive decline is inherent to the aging process, the trajectory with which this decline occurs presents enormous inter and intra-individual variability, as a consequence of the influence of multiple factors with potential modulating effect. First, the progressive increase in average life expectancy, as a result of advances in medicine and better living conditions, implies differentiated functional and clinical contexts in the various age groups of the older population, which will determine important functional differences in cognition. On the other hand, chronic diseases that affect the cardiovascular system, such as diabetes, hypertension and dyslipidemia, among others, not only increase in prevalence with age, but also contribute to accelerate the cognitive decline of the individual. The impact of aging on cognition will thus express the individual genetic heritage and the result of its interaction with the environment, resulting in very marked patterns of inter-individual variability, but also trends in intra-individual variability in the face of circumstantially determining events that could modify the biological aging process. Aspects such as literacy, culture, health status, life experiences, ethnicity, socioeconomic status, emotional factors and motivation, among others, are also important sources of variability in individual trajectories of cognitive decline as a function of age, so that these trajectories, rather than translating a linear relationship, express a dynamic and mutable process. An example of this dynamic nature of the trajectory of cognitive function with age stems from the results of the ACTIVE study, which analyzed the benefits of cognitive training in a cohort of older people, demonstrating benefits in terms of overall cognitive performance, and revealing the preservation of neural plasticity in the older adult, allowing for the optimization of their cognitive performance and learning of new skills or abilities[39]. Moreover, this trajectory of cognitive decline varies depending on the cognitive function considered, where some aspects decline linearly with age, while other aspects remain stable until later stages of life, at which time a marked functional decline occurs. Consideration must be given to the limited ecological value of many cognitive function assessment tools, on the one hand, and the ability of many old adults to maintain high levels of competence in daily activities by the ability to compensate for cognitive decline with the accumulated experience.

Strategies for promoting a healthy cognitive aging

One of the fundamental challenges in view of the demographic trend of modern societies is the promotion of healthy and active aging through strategies aimed at preventing the decline that accompanies biological senescence. The identification and implementation of programs that positively modulate cognitive function in the older adult should be a priority programmatic axis, given the importance of cognition in the daily routine of the individual. In this sense, several interventions have been tested, with particular emphasis on issues directly related to lifestyles. In fact, there is a scientifically grounded belief[40,41] that an active lifestyle and involvement in certain everyday activities can contribute to the prevention of cognitive decline associated with aging. Properly tailored physical exercise and active daily activities (e.g., gardening and dancing) are recognized as beneficial for cognition, as well as engaging in intellectually stimulating activities such as chess, puzzles, reading, musical practice, among others[42]. These aspects positively modulate cognitive reserve by optimizing neural plasticity, so that the individual's level of cognitive function reflects the balance between the magnitude of brain changes due to aging and the ability of the same brain to compensate for these changes through its cognitive reserve.

Several studies have provided robust results supporting the importance of physical and intellectual activity in cognitive function. A previously cited example, the ACTIVE study, has shown the cognitive benefits of cognitive training in a cohort of older people[39]. A recent meta-analysis of prospective cohort studies has shown a reduction in the risk of dementia in people engaged in vigorous physical activity[43]. In another study, a three-month period of aerobic exercise was associated with improvements in attention, memory, and executive functions[44], while other studies identified cognitive benefits accompanied by changes in brain structure, including bilateral increase in anterior hippocampal volume[45]. Involvement in social activities, such as socializing with family and friends and participating in cultural events, has also been shown to promote better cognitive function in the older adult.

Another key aspect in preventing cognitive decline associated with aging is nutrition. In fact, nutritional factors such as calorie and macro and micronutrient intake greatly influence brain function during the aging process. Calorie restriction has been historically recognized as a beneficial strategy for maintaining health and well-being, having implications on aging biology. The mechanisms inherent to this benefit have been widely studied, with particular emphasis on nutrient signaling pathways that act upon the detection of circulating nutrient variations or intracellular metabolites indicating energy metabolism[46]. These axes play a major role in the biology of aging and are closely linked to aspects such as oxidative stress, gene expression, vascular inflammation and pathology, apoptosis and mitochondrial function. On the other hand, the optimization of brain function depends on a close balance between macro and micronutrients[47], hence any nutritional-based strategy for promoting a healthy cognitive aging will necessarily have to fit the individual needs and be applied in a personalized perspective. The AGA@4life model embodies this multidisciplinary and personalized approach to promoting healthy aging, focusing on the individual needs, and tailoring the intervention plans at the nutritional level, among other dimensions such as physical exercise. Indeed, the results of the pilot implementation of this intervention model have demonstrated significant benefits in the cognitive function of older people, particularly in terms of motor control, processing speed, SWM, learning and visuospatial capacity[48]. These results identify the AGA@4life Model as an effective non-pharmacological instrument for positively modulating the pathways of cognitive decline in the older adult, particularly when implemented in a personalized approach and within a multi-componential framework.

Conclusion

The neurobiology of aging marks a progressive decline in certain cognitive dimensions, such as processing speed, memory, executive functions, learning, among others. Given the potential impact of these modifications, it is imperative to develop intervention strategies that promote or preserve cognition as part of comprehensive programs to promote healthy aging. The implementation of a comprehensive intervention program, as advocated in the AGA@4life model, incorporating physical activity, nutritional counseling, promotion of social interaction and cognitive stimulation tailored to the individual needs, provides a consistent and effective opportunity to modulate the pathway of lifelong functional decline in a more favorable sense. In fact, recent data support the AGA@4life intervention model as an effective non-pharmacological tool for positive cognitive modulation in older people, based on a personalized approach and multi-component structure, with demonstrated benefits in processing speed and motor control, memory and learning[48].

Key points

- Decline in cognitive function in aging is a common and extremely heterogeneous process.
- Structural and functional changes that occur in the brain with aging determine the trajectory of cognitive decline.
- Implementation of approaches to preserve or promote good cognitive function in aging should be a strategic priority.
- Intervention programs aimed at neurocognitive protection should be personalized, multidisciplinary, and systematic.
- The AGA@4life Model is an effective non-pharmacological tool for positive cognitive modulation in older people.

References

1 World Health Organization (WHO). Number of people over 60 years set to double by 2015; major societal changes required. Media centre. News Release, World Health Organization, 2015.

2　Instituto Nacional de Estatística. Envelhecimento da população residente em Portugal e na União Europeia. Lisboa: INE; 2015.

3　Lutz W, Sanderson W, Scherbov S. The coming acceleration of global population ageing. Nature. 2008;451:716–9.

3　Gilbert SF. Developmental biology. 6th edition. Sunderland, MA: Sinauer Associates; 2000.

4　Terry RD, Katzman R. Life span and synapses: will there be a primary senile dementia? Neurobiol Aging. 2001;22:347–8.

5　Raz N, Gunning-Dixon FM, Head D, Dupuis JH, Acker JD. Neuroanatomical correlates of cognitive aging: evidence from structural magnetic resonance imaging. Neuropsychology. 1998;12:95–114.

6　Raz N, Rodrigue KM, Head D, Kennedy KM, Acker JD. Differential aging of the medial temporal lobe: a study of a five-year change. Neurology. 2004;62:433–8.

7　Uttara B, Singh AV, Zamboni P, Mahajan RT. Oxidative stress and neurodegenerative diseases: a review of upstream and downstream antioxidant therapeutic options. Curr Neuropharmacol. 2009;7:65–74.

8　Terry RD, Katzman R. Life span and synapses: will there be a primary senile dementia? Neurobiol Aging. 2001;22:347–8.

9　Resnick SM, Pham DL, Kraut MA, Zonderman AB, Davatzikos C. Longitudinal magnetic resonance imaging studies of older adults: a shrinking brain. J Neurosci: Official J Soc Neurosci. 2003;23:3295–301.

10　Dickstein DL, Kabaso D, Rocher AB, Luebke JI, Wearne SL, Hof PR. Changes in the structural complexity of the aged brain. Aging Cell. 2007;6:275–84.

11　Dumitriu D, Hao J, Hara Y, Kaufmann J, Janssen WG, Lou W, Rapp PR, Morrison JH. Selective changes in thin spine density and morphology in monkey prefrontal cortex correlate with aging-related cognitive impairment. J Neurosci. 2010;30(22):7507–15.

12　Navarro-Martinez R, Fernandez-Garrido J, Buigues C, Torralba-Martinez E, Martinez-Martinez M, Verdejo Y, Mascaros MC, Cauli O. Brain-derived neurotrophic factor correlates with functional and cognitive impairment in non-disabled older individuals. Exp Gerontol. 2015;72:129–37.

13　Ryan MM, Guevremont D, Luxmanan C, Abraham WC, Williams JM. Aging alters long-term potentiation–related gene networks and impairs synaptic protein synthesis in the rat hippocampus. Neurobiol Aging. 2015;36:1868–80.

14　Johnson DA, Johnson JA. Nrf2—a therapeutic target for the treatment of neurodegenerative diseases. Free Radic Biol Med. 2015;88:253–67.

15　Hara Y, Punsoni M, Yuk F, Park CS, Janssen WG, Rapp PR, Morrison JH. Synaptic distributions of GluA2 and PKMzeta in the monkey dentate gyrus and their relationships with aging and memory. J Neurosci. 2012;32(21):7336–44.

16　Robbins TW, Arnsten AF. The neuropsychopharmacology of fronto-executive function: monoaminergic modulation. Annu Rev Neurosci. 2009;32:267–87.

17 Pike KE, Savage G, Villemagne VL, et al. Beta-amyloid imaging and memory in non-demented individuals: evidence for preclinical Alzheimer's disease. Brain J Neurol. 2007;130:2837–44.

18 Jack CR Jr, Lowe VJ, Senjem ML, et al. 11C PiB and structural MRI provide complementary information in imaging of Alzheimer's disease and amnestic mild cognitive impairment. Brain J Neurol. 2008;131:665–80.

19 Salat DH, Kaye JA, Janowsky JS. Prefrontal gray and white matter volumes in healthy aging and Alzheimer disease. Arch Neurol. 1999;56:338–44.

20 Meier-Ruge W, Ulrich J, Bruhlmann M, Meier E. Age-related white matter atrophy in the human brain. Ann N Y Acad Sci. 1992;673:260–9.

21 Rogalski E, Stebbins GT, Barnes CA, et al. Age-related changes in parahippocampal white matter integrity: a diffusion tensor imaging study. Neuropsychologia. 2012;50:1759–65.

22 Salthouse TA. Selective review of cognitive aging. J Int Neuropsychol Soc. 2010;16:754–60.

23 Haaland KY, Price L, Larue A. What does the WMS-III tell us about memory changes with normal aging? J Int Neuropsychol Soc. 2003;9:89–96.

24 Whiting WL 4th, Smith AD. Differential age-related processing limitations in recall and recognition tasks. Psychol Aging. 1997;12:216–24.

25 Ronnlund M, Nyberg L, Backman L, Nilsson LG. Stability, growth, and decline in adult life span development of declarative memory: cross-sectional and longitudinal data from a population-based study. Psychol Aging. 2005;20:3–18.

26 Hedden T, Gabrieli JD. Insights into the ageing mind: a view from cognitive neuroscience. Nat Rev Neurosci. 2004;5:87–96.

27 Isingrini M, Taconnat L. Episodic memory, frontal functioning, and aging. Rev Neurol. 2008;164(Suppl 3):S91–5.

28 Davis HP, Klebe KJ, Guinther PM, Schroder KB, Cornwell RE, James LE. Subjective organization, verbal learning, and forgetting across the life span: from 5 to 89. Exp Aging Res. 2013;39:1–26.

29 Zacks RT, Hasher L, Li KZH. Human memory. In: Craik FI, Salthouse TA (eds.), The handbook of aging and cognition. 2nd edition. Mahwah, NJ: Erlbaum; 2000. pp. 293–357.

30 Salthouse TA, Fristoe NM, Lineweaver TT, Coon VE. Aging of attention: does the ability to divide decline? Mem Cognit. 1995;23:59–71.

31 Carlson MC, Hasher L, Zacks RT, Connelly SL. Aging, distraction, and the benefits of predictable location. Psychol Aging. 1995;10:427–36.

32 Carriere JS, Cheyne JA, Solman GJ, Smilek D. Age trends for failures of sustained attention. Psychol Aging. 2010;25(3):569–74.

33 Singh-Manoux A, Kivimaki M, Glymour MM, et al. Timing of onset of cognitive decline: results from Whitehall II prospective cohort study. BMJ. 2012;344:d7622.

34 Zec RF, Markwell SJ, Burkett NR, Larsen DL. A longitudinal study of confrontation naming in the "normal" elderly. J Int Neuropsychol Soc. 2005;11:716–26.

35 Weber M, Wu T, Hanson JE, Alam NM, Solanoy H, Ngu H, Lauffer BE, Lin HH, Dominguez SL, Reeder J, Tom J, Steiner P, Foreman O, Prusky GT, Scearce-Levie K. Cognitive deficits, changes in synaptic function, and brain pathology in a mouse model of normal aging(1,2,3). eNeuro. 2015;2(5):ENEURO.0047-15.2015.

36 Stokes MG. 'Activity-silent' working memory in prefrontal cortex: a dynamic coding framework. Trends Cogn Sci. 2015;19:394–40.

37 Robbins T, James M, Owen A, Sahakian BJ, Mclnnes L, et al. Cambridge Neuropsychological Test Automated Battery (CANTAB): a factor analytic study of a large sample of normal elderly volunteers. Dementia. 1994;5:266–81.

38 Robbins T, James M, Owen A, Sahakian BJ, Lawrence AD, et al. A study of performance on tests from the CANTAB battery sensitive to frontal lobe dysfunction in a large sample of normal volunteers: implications for theories of executive functioning and cognitive aging. J Int Neuropsychol Soc. 1998;4:474–90.

39 Ball K, Berch DB, Helmers KF, Jobe JB, Leveck MD, Marsiske M, Morris JN, Rebok GW, Smith DM, Tennstedt SL, Unverzagt FW, Willis SL. Effects of cognitive training interventions with older adults: a randomized controlled trial. JAMA. 2002;288(18):2271–81.

40 Marioni RE, van den Hout A, Valenzuela MJ, et al. Active cognitive lifestyle associates with cognitive recovery and a reduced risk of cognitive decline. J Alzheimer's Dis. 2012;28:223–30.

41 Fratiglioni L, Paillard-Borg S, Winblad B. An active and socially integrated lifestyle in late life might protect against dementia. Lancet Neurol. 2004;3:343–53.

42 Verghese J, Lipton RB, Katz MJ, et al. Leisure activities and the risk of dementia in the elderly. N Engl J Med. 2003;348:2508–16.

43 Guure CB, Ibrahim NA, Adam MB, Said SM. Impact of physical activity on cognitive decline, dementia, and its subtypes: meta-analysis of prospective studies. Biomed Res Int. 2017;2017:9016924.

44 Barnes DE, Santos-Modesitt W, Poelke G, Kramer AF, Castro C, Middleton LE, Yaffe K. The Mental Activity and eXercise (MAX) trial: a randomized controlled trial to enhance cognitive function in older adults. JAMA Intern Med. 2013;173(9):797–804.

45 Erickson KI, Raji CA, Lopez OL, Becker JT, Rosano C, Newman AB, Gach HM, Thompson PM, Ho AJ, Kuller LH. Physical activity predicts gray matter volume in late adulthood: the Cardiovascular Health Study. Neurology. 2010;75(16):1415–22.

46 Koubova J, Guarente L. How does calorie restriction work? Genes Dev. 2003;17:313–21.

47 Mallidou A, Cartie M. Nutritional habits and cognitive performance of older adults. Nurs Manag (Harrow). 2015;22:27–34.

48 Pereira T, Cipriano I, Costa T, Saraiva M, Martins A, in behalf of the AGA@4life Consortium. Exercise, ageing and cognitive function – effects of a personalized physical exercise program in the cognitive function of older adults. Physiol Behav. 2019;202:8–13.

Index

Abordagem Geriátrica Ampla (AGA) 83
absolute intensity 28
active aging 83, 119
ACTIVE study 155–156
adherence management 86
adherence to therapy 84–85
AGA@4life intervention model 4–5, 6, 33, 119–120, 126–127; beneficial effect of pharmacological counseling on hepatic steatosis 145–146; described 4; role of 136–137; steps of 5; and therapeutic management of older adult 86–87
age-associated changes: in cholesterol homeostasis 103–104; in cholesterol metabolism cardiovascular risk 99–108; and exercise effect on lipid profile 99–108
aging: active 83, 119; benefits of exercise for 32; causes of 58; clinical manifestations 116; cognitive function and 149–157; defined 24, 90; effects on the body 116–117; and health care costs 24; and liver changes 142; and liver steatosis 145; and malnutrition 57; muscle 117; musculoskeletal ultrasound and 118; nutrition in 56–63; physiological changes 25–28; and polymedication 142–143; Portuguese population 56–567; structural changes resulting from 116

aging brain 149–151; additional changes in 151
aging heart 124–126; AGA@4life intervention model 126–127; arterial changes 126; changes in heart function 125–126; changes in heart valves 124–125; structural and functional changes of 124–128
aging process 114–115, 141–142; biological dimension 115; and cholesterol metabolism 103; and cognitive function decline 154–156; progressive 115; psychological dimension 115; singular 115; social dimension 115; vascular 134
air quality: defined 65; indoor 65
American College of Sports Medicine 29–30
arterial aging 130–133; and AGA@4life intervention model 136–137; determinants of early vascular aging 135–136; early vascular aging (EVA) 133–135; positive modulators of arterial function 136–137; see also aging
arterial changes 126
arterial hypertension (AH) 132, 134, 136–137
Ascension 26
atherosclerosis 134
ATP-binding cassette (ABC) transporters 102
atrophy 26

attention: cognitive function 152; divided 152; selective 91, 152
auditory training: effect in the older adult's lives 90–96; filtered speech test 92; sentences test with ipsilateral competitive message 93; speech in noise test 92–93
autonomic nervous system (ANS) 43–46

balance 12–13; and mobility 13; static 13
Bandura, A. 13
BDNF (brain derived neurotrophic factor) 150
Beier, L.O. 95
Bellis, T. 91
bicompartmental model 25
biofeedback 16
body: effects of aging on 116–117; and muscle aging 117
body composition 25
BrainAnswer: comparison of HRV parameters of old and young participant 43–50; described 37; experimental design 38–43; and heart rate variability (HRV) analysis metrics 38; IPAQ results 50–**52**, *51*; methods for testing 38; for older adults 36–53; testing 38–43

Cambridge Neuropsychological Test Automated Battery (CANTAB – Cambridge Cognition, Cambridge, UK) 154
carbon dioxide (CO_2): average concentration of 71–74, **71–74**; described 66; in indoor air 75
carbon monoxide (CO): average concentration of 71–74, **71–74**; below protection threshold value 75; described 66
cardiorespiratory capacity 26
Carvalho, C.R. 90
Central Auditory Processing (CAP) 90–92
central nervous system 27
cholesterol: biosynthesis 100–102; and cardiovascular risk in older patients 104–106; high density lipoprotein (HDL) 100, 105, 107; low-density lipoprotein (LDL) 100, 103–105, 107–108; metabolism of 99–103
cholesterol ester transfer protein (CETP) 106–107
cholesterol homeostasis 100; age-associated changes in 103–104
cholesterol metabolism cardiovascular risk 99–108
chronic noncommunicable diseases 84
cognitive aging, strategies for promoting a healthy 155–157
cognitive function: and aging 151–153; aging brain 149–151; attention 152; executive functions 152–153; language 153; memory 151–152; processing speed 151; study in the older adult 153–154; variability of decline in older adult 154–155; visuospatial capacity 153
comprehensive geriatric approach (AGA): advantages of 3–4; described 2; dimensions and subdimensions of *3*; structure 2–3
Correia P. 26
Cury, M.C.L. 91

declarative (explicit) memory 152
demographic aging 149; challenges 1–2; in Portugal 114; solutions to problems of 2–4, *3*; *see also* aging
diagnosis of structural changes in human body 117–118
diagnostic-intervention continuum 2
Dias, G. 24
divided attention 152
dual energy radiographic absorptiometry (DEXA) 117

early vascular aging (EVA) 133–135; determinants of **133**, 135–136
electrocardiogram (ECG) signal 38; acquired, of participants *44*; display, of participants *45*

Energy Certification System (ECS) 68–69
environmental pollutants **67**; *see also specific types*
episodic (autobiographical) memory 152
European Group for the Study of Sarcopenia 61
European Society of Hypertension 132
European Systematic Coronary Risk Assessment (SCORE) dataset 105
executive functions 152–153
exercise: based intervention programs 15–17; effect on lipid profile 99–108; and functional ability 10; and healthy aging 10–11; older adult with chronic disease 30–32, **31**; physical, applied to older people 24–33; self-efficacy for 13–15; and serum lipids 106–108
experimental design: BrainAnswer 38–43; data acquisition *42*, 42–43; data treatment 43; equipment 40–42, *41–42*; protocol 39; sensor placement procedures 39–40; target population 39

falls: defined 10; and muscle strength 12; and older adults 10; programs for the prevention of 13–15; reducing, in older adults 10; risk screening 11–13
FallSensing system 2
Ferreira, A. 75
filtered speech test 92
flexibility training 30
Forced Expiratory Volume in 1 second (FEV_1) 26
Forced Vital Capacity (FVC) 26
formaldehyde (CH_2O) 66–68; average concentration of 71–74, **71–74**
Frank–Starling mechanism 126
frequency domain analysis of HRV parameters 46–**50**, *47*, **48**, *49*
functional assessment 11–13; improving functioning 11–12; muscle strength 12

Functional Fitness Test 30
Functional Residual Capacity (CRF) 26

Global Strategy and Action Plan for Ageing and Health 9
Golgi Complex apparatus 101
Gonçales, A.S. 91
Guarinello, A.C. 90

handgrip strength 11–12
health: benefits of exercise for 32; effects of environmental pollutants on **67**
healthy aging: and exercise 10–11; overview 9; strategies for 9–17; *see also* aging
hearing loss 27
heart function, changes in 125–126
heart rate variability (HRV) analysis metrics 38; comparison of old and young participants 43–50; frequency domain analysis of 46–**50**, *47*, **48**, *49*; nonlinear HRV parameters 50; time domain analysis of 46
heart valves, changes in 124–125
Hemodynamic Aging Syndrome 134
hepatic characterization of senior population and its relationship with polymedication 141–146
hepatic impairment 143–144
hepatic steatosis: and AGA@4life intervention program 145; beneficial effect of pharmacological counseling on 145–146; nonalcoholic 107
high density lipoprotein (HDL) cholesterol 100, 105, 107
Home Safety Checklist for Fall Prevention 15
human body: diagnosis of structural changes in 117–118
HVAC systems rulles 69
hydration 62

Índice de Complexidade da Farmacoterapia (ICFT) 86–87

individualized nutritional
intervention 61
indoor air: evaluation and older
people 65–79; and health effects
66; pollution 68
indoor air quality (IAQ) 65;
evaluation 69–77; and health
effects 66; materials and methods
of evaluation 69–70; results of
evaluation 71–74, **71–74**
International Classification
qualifiers of Functioning,
Disability and Health (ICF) 10
International Physical Activity
Questionnaire (IPAQ) 38; results
50–**52**, *51*
intervention programs 119–120;
AGA@4life project 119–120; and
biofeedback 16; exercise-based
15–17; Otago Exercise Program
(OTAGO) 15–16; physical activity
119; and their benefits 119–120

Jani, B. 135
Jesus, L. 75
Jones, B. A. 30

kinesthesia 27

language, as cognitive function
153
lean mass 25
lipid profile: exercise effect on
99–108; maternal 107
liver changes and aging 142
liver evaluation, ultrasound as a
method of 144–145
liver steatosis: and aging 145; and
polymedication 145
Loureiro, A. 75
low-density lipoprotein (LDL)
cholesterol 100, 103–105, 107–108

malnutrition: and aging 57; causes
in older people 57; MNA for identifying risk of 59; prevention and
treatment of 57; results, in older
people 59
Martínez-Gómez, D. 11
Martins, J. 92
Martins, L. 75

Masugata, H. 125
maternal lipid profile 107
medication adherence 85
Medication Regimen Complexity
Index (MRCI) 86–87
memory: cognitive function
151–152; declarative (explicit) 152;
episodic (autobiographical)
152; non-declarative (implicit)
152; short-term 152; working
150, 152
metabolism of cholesterol 99–103
micronutrients 62
Mini-Mental State Examination 154
Mini Nutritional Assessment (MNA)
58–59
mobility: and balance 13; Step test
13
Mobility-related Activity and
Participation Profile (PAPM)
9–10
Montreal Cognitive Assessment
Battery (MOCA) 154
motivation, and self-efficacy 13–14
Motor Screening Task (MOT) 154
multidisciplinary intervention
program: impact on skeletal
muscle in older adult 114–120
muscle aging 117
muscle thickness (MT): defined
118; increasing 120; and muscle
strength 118
muscle ultrasound assessment 118
musculoskeletal system 26–27
musculoskeletal ultrasound and
aging 118

nanoparticles 68; average
concentration of 71–74, **71–74**
National Energy Certification
System 68
National Institute of Statistics (INE)
114
neuroscientific research 149
Niemann-Pick C1Like 1 protein
(NPC1L1) 102
noncommunicable diseases 84
non-declarative (implicit) memory
152
nonlinear HRV parameters
50

nutrition: in aging 56–63; maintaining proper 61–62; nutritional status assessment 59–61; screening 58–59

nutritional needs 61–62

nutritional risk screening 58–59

nutritional status assessment 59–61

obesity 60

older adult: AGA@4life model and therapeutic management of 86–87; and auditory training 90–96; BrainAnswer platform for 36–53; with chronic disease 30–32, **31**; and indoor air evaluation 65–79; malnutrition causes in 57; modulators and determinants of arterial aging in 130–138; multidisciplinary intervention program and skeletal muscle in 114–120; nutritional needs 61–62; nutritional status assessment 60; and physical exercise 24–33; polymedicated 83–88; polymedication in 84; positive modulators of arterial function in 136–137; study of cognitive function in 153–154; variability of cognitive function decline in 154–155; without chronic disease 29–30

older patients: cholesterol and cardiovascular risk in 104–106

older people *see* older adult

Otago Exercise Program (OTAGO) 15–16

outcome expectations 14

Paired Associates Learning (PAL) 154

pharmacological counseling: beneficial effect on hepatic steatosis 145–146; on hepatic steatosis 145–146

pharmacological treatment: adherence to therapy 84–85; AGA@4life model and therapeutic management of older adult 86–87; and polymedicated older adult 83–88; polymedication in older adult 84; therapeutic complexity 85–86

physical activity 119

physical exercise: defined 28; levels 28–29; and older people 24–33; recommendations 29–30; *see also* exercise

physiological changes: aging 25–28; body composition 25; cardiorespiratory capacity 26; central nervous system 27; musculoskeletal system 26–27; sensory and perceptual system 27–28

$PM_{2.5}$ fine particles 68; average concentration of 71–74, **71–74**, 76

PM_{10} coarse particles 68; average concentration of 71–74, **71–74**, 76

polymedicated older adult: pharmacological treatment and 83–88

polymedication: aging and 142–143; and hepatic characterization of senior population 141–146; and liver steatosis 145; in the older adult 84

population aging 90; as social and economic problem 1

Portugal: aging index 56–57; aging process 114–115; demographic aging in 114; population and aging 56–57

positive modulators of arterial function in older adult 136–137

processing speed 151

proprioception 27

quality of life 62

Rajkumar, C. 135

Rapid Visual Information Processing 154

Reaction Time (RTI) 154

relative intensity 28

Renner, B. 14

Residual Volume (VR) 26

Rikli, R. E. 30

sarcopenia 61, 117

Schwarzer, R. 14

SDNN index 46

sedentary behavior 11

selective attention 91, 152

self-efficacy: assessment 14; beliefs 14; defined 13; for exercise 13–15; and motivation 13–14
Self-efficacy for Exercise Scale 14
sensory and perceptual system 27–28
sentences test with ipsilateral competitive message 93
serum lipids: effect of exercise on 106–108
short-term memory 152
Sick Building Syndrome (SED) 68
Silva A. 26
Spatial Working Memory (SWM) 154
speech in noise test 92–93
static balance 13
Step test 13
Sterol Sensing Domain (SSD) 101
strategies for promoting a healthy cognitive aging 155–157
study of cognitive function in older adult 153–154
sympathetic nervous system 46
sympathovagal balance 46

Telephone Interview for Cognitive Status 154
TG-rich lipoproteins 107
therapeutic complexity 85–86
therapy: adherence to 84–85; therapeutic complexity 85–86
30 Seconds Sit to Stand test 12
Thomas Sydenham aphorism 130

Tiffeneau Index (IT) 26
time domain analysis of HRV parameters 46
Timed Up and Go (TUG) test 12
total cholesterol (TC) 100, 104–105
triglycerides (TG) 100; content 107; hydrolysis 107; levels 107; reserves 106
The 2012 Aging Report Economic and budgetary projections for the 27 EU Member States (2010–2060) 36

ultrasound: as a method of liver evaluation 144–145; muscle ultrasound assessment 118; musculoskeletal 118
United Nations 124

Vellas, B. 59
vision 27
visuospatial capacity 153

Warren, Marjory 2
working memory 150, 152
World Health Organization (WHO) 9, 15, 28, 29, 30, 32, 83, 85, 115, 119, 124; on indoor air pollution 68; on indoor air quality and health effects 66; quality of life 62; Sick Building Syndrome (SED) 68
World Population Prospects – The 2015 Revision report 124

Printed in the United States
by Baker & Taylor Publisher Services